Current Clinical Strategies

Pediatric History and Physical Examination

Fourth Edition

Elizabeth K. Albright, MD

Current Clinical Strategies Publishing
www.ccspublishing.com/ccs

Digital Book and Updates

Purchasers of this book can download the digital book and updates at the Current Clinical Strategies Publishing Internet site: www.ccspublishing.com/ccs

Current Clinical Strategies Publishing
27071 Cabot Road
Laguna Hills, California 92653-7011
Phone: 800-331-8227
Fax: 800-965-9420
E-mail: info@ccspublishing.com
Internet: www.ccspublishing.com/ccs

Printed in USA   ISBN 1881528-92-8

Contents

Medical Documentation

Pediatric History

Identifying Data: Patient's name, age, sex; significant medical conditions, informant (parent).

Chief Compliant (CC): Reason that the child is seeking medical care and duration of the symptom.

History of Present Illness (HPI): Describe the course of the patient's illness, including when and how it began, character of the symptoms; aggravating or alleviating factors; pertinent positives and negatives, past diagnostic testing.

Past Medical History (PMH): Medical problems, hospitalizations, operations; asthma, diabetes.

Perinatal History: Gestational age at birth, obstetrical complications, type of delivery, birth weight, Apgar scores, complications (eg, infection, jaundice), length of hospital stay.

Medications: Names and dosages.

Nutrition: Type of diet, amount taken each feed, change in feeding habits.

Developmental History: Age at attainment of important milestones (walking, talking, self-care). Relationships with siblings, peers, adults. School grade and performance, behavioral problems.

Immunizations: Up-to-date?

Allergies: Penicillin, codeine?

Family History: Medical problems in family, including the patient's disorder; diabetes, seizures, asthma, allergies, cancer, cardiac, renal or GI disease, tuberculosis, smoking.

Social History: Family situation, alcohol, smoking, drugs, sexual activity. Parental level of education. Safety: Child car seats, smoke detectors, bicycle helmets.

Review of Systems (ROS)

General: Overall health, weight loss, behavioral changes, fever, fatigue.

Skin: Rashes, moles, bruising, lumps/bumps, nail/hair changes.

Eyes: Visual problems, eye pain.

Ear, nose, throat: Frequency of colds, pharyngitis, otitis media.

Lungs: Cough, shortness of breath, wheezing.

Cardiovascular: Chest pain, murmurs, syncope.

Gastrointestinal: Nausea/vomiting, spitting up, diarrhea, recurrent abdominal pain, constipation, blood in stools.

Genitourinary: Dysuria, hematuria, polyuria, vaginal discharge, STDs.

Musculoskeletal: Weakness, joint pain, gait abnormalities, scoliosis.

Neurological: Headache, seizures.

Endocrine: Growth delay, polyphagia, excessive thirst/fluid intake, menses duration, amount of flow.

Pediatric Physical Examination

Observation: Child's facial expression (pain), response to social overtures. Interaction with caretakers and examiner. Body position (leaning forward in sitting position; epiglottitis, pericarditis). Weak cry (serious illness), high-pitched cry (increased intracranial pressure, metabolic disorder); moaning (serious illness, meningitis), grunting (respiratory distress).

Does the child appear to be:
(1) Well, acutely ill/toxic, chronically ill, wasted, or malnourished?
(2) Alert and active or lethargic/fatigued?
(3) Well hydrated or dehydrated?
(4) Unusual body odors?

Vital Signs: Respiratory rate, blood pressure, pulse, temperature.

Measurements: Height, weight; head circumference in children ≤2 years; plot on growth charts and determine growth percentiles.

Skin: Cyanosis, jaundice, pallor, rashes, skin turgor, edema, hemangiomas, café au lait spots, nevi, Mongolian spots, hair distribution, capillary refill (in seconds).

Lymph Nodes: Location, size, tenderness, mobility and consistency of cervical, axillary, supraclavicular, and inguinal nodes.

Head: Size, shape, asymmetry, cephalohematoma, bossing, molding, bruits, fontanelles (size, tension), dilated veins, facial asymmetry.

Eyes: Pupils equal round and reactive to light and accommodation (PERRLA); extraocular movements intact (EOMI); Brushfield's spots; epicanthic folds, discharge, conjunctiva; red reflex, corneal opacities, cataracts, fundi; strabismus (eye deviation); visual acuity.

Ears: Pinnas (position, size), tympanic membranes (landmarks, mobility, erythema, dull, shiny, bulging), hearing.

Nose: Shape, discharge, bleeding, mucosa, patency.

Mouth: Lips (thinness, downturning, fissures, cleft lip), teeth, mucus membrane color and moisture (enanthem, Epstein's pearls), tongue, cleft palate.

Throat: Tonsils (erythema, exudate), postnasal drip, hoarseness, stridor.

Neck: Torticollis, lymphadenopathy, thyroid nodules, position of trachea.

Thorax: Shape, symmetry, intercostal or substernal retractions.

Breasts: Turner stage, size, shape, symmetry, masses, nipple discharge, gynecomastia.

Lungs: Breathing rate, depth, expansion, prolongation of expiration, fremitus, dullness to percussion, breath sounds, crackles, wheezing, rhonchi.

Heart: Location of apical impulse. Regular rate and rhythm (RRR), first and second heart sounds (S1, S2); gallops (S3, S4), murmurs (location, position in cycle, intensity grade 1-6, pitch, effect of change of position, transmission). Comparison of brachial and femoral pulses.

Abdomen: Contour, visible peristalsis, respiratory movements, dilated veins, umbilicus, bowel sounds, bruits, hernia. Rebound tenderness, tympany; hepatomegaly, splenomegaly, masses.

Genitalia:
  Male Genitalia: Circumcision, hypospadias, phimosis, size of testes, cryptorchidism, hydrocele, hernia, inguinal masses.
  Female Genitalia: Imperforate hymen, discharge, labial adhesions, clitoral hypertrophy, pubertal changes.

Rectum and Anus: Erythema, excoriation, fissures, prolapse, imperforate anus. Anal tone, masses, tenderness, anal reflex.

Extremities: Bow legs (infancy), knock knees (age 2 to 3 years). Edema (grade 1-4+), cyanosis, clubbing. Joint range of motion, swelling, redness, tenderness. A "click" felt on rotation of hips indicates developmental hip dislocation (Barlow maneuver). Extra digits, simian lines, pitting of nails, flat feet.

Spine and Back: Scoliosis, rigidity, pilonidal dimple, pilonidal cyst, sacral hair tufts; tenderness over spine or costovertebral tenderness.

Neurological Examination:

  Behavior: Level of consciousness, intelligence, emotional status.

  Motor system: Gait, muscle tone, strength (graded 0 to 5).

  Reflexes

   Deep Tendon Reflexes: Biceps, brachioradialis, triceps, patellar, and Achilles reflexes (graded 1-4).

   Superficial Reflexes: Abdominal, cremasteric, plantar reflexes

   Neonatal Reflexes: Babinski, Landau, Moro, rooting, suck, grasp, tonic neck reflexes.

Developmental Assessment: Delayed abilities for age on developmental screening test.

Laboratory Evaluation: Electrolytes (sodium, potassium, bicarbonate, chloride, BUN, creatinine), CBC (hemoglobin, hematocrit, WBC count, platelets, differential); X-rays, urinalysis (UA).

Assessment: Assign a number to each problem, and discuss each problem separately. Discuss the differential diagnosis, and give reasons that support the working diagnosis. Give reasons for excluding other diagnoses.

Plan: Describe therapeutic plan for each numbered problem, including testing, laboratory studies, medications, antibiotics, and consultations.

Physical Examination of the Newborn

General Appearance: Overall visual and auditory appraisal of the completely undressed infant. Weak cry (serious illness), high-pitched cry (increased intracranial pressure, metabolic disorders), grunting (respiratory distress). Unusual body odors.

Vital Signs: Respiratory rate (normal 40-60 breaths/min), heart rate (120-160 beats/minute), temperature.

Head: Lacerations, caput, cephalohematoma, skull molding. Fontanelles (size, tension), head circumference.

Neck: Flexibility and asymmetry.

Eyes: Scleral hemorrhages, cataracts, red reflex, pupil size.

Mouth: Palpate for cleft lip and cleft palate.

Respiratory: Acrocyanosis, retractions, nasal flaring, grunting. Palpation of clavicles for fractures.

Heart: Position of point of maximal impulse, rhythm, murmurs. Distant heart sounds (pneumothorax). Comparison of brachial and femoral pulses.

Abdomen: Asymmetry, masses, fullness, umbilicus, hernias. Liver span (may extend 2.5 cm below the right costal margin), spleen span, nephromegaly.

Male Genitalia: Hypospadias, phimosis, hernia, presence of both testes. Anal patency

Female Genitalia: Interlabial masses, mucoid vaginal discharge or blood streaked discharge (normal). Anal patency

Skin: Pink, cyanotic, pale. Jaundice (abnormal in the first day of life), milia (yellow papules), Mongolian spots (bluish patches).

Extremities: Extra digits, simian lines, pilonidal dimple or cyst, sacral hair tuft, hip dislocation; a "click" felt on rotation of hips (Barlow maneuver, developmental hip dislocation).

Neurologic Examination: Tone, activity, symmetry of extremity movement, symmetry of facial movements, alertness, consolability, Moro reflex, suck reflex, root reflex, grasp reflex, plantar reflex.

Progress Notes

Daily progress notes should summarize developments in the patient's hospital course, problems that remain active, plans to treat those problems, and arrangements for discharge. Progress notes should address every problem on the problem list.

Example Progress Note

Date/time:
Subjective: Any problems and symptoms should be charted. Appetite, pain or fussiness may be included.
Objective:
  General appearance.
  Vitals, temperature, maximum temperature over past 24 hours, pulse, respiratory rate, blood pressure. Feedings, fluid I/O (inputs and outputs), daily weights.
  Physical exam, including chest and abdomen, with particular attention to active problems. Emphasize changes from previous physical exams.
Laboratory Evaluation: New test results. Circle abnormal values.
Current medications: List medications and dosages.
Assessment and Plan: This section should be organized by problem. A separate assessment and plan should be written for each problem.

Discharge Note

The discharge note should be written prior to discharge.

Discharge Note

Date/time:
Diagnoses:
Treatment: Briefly describe therapy provided during hospitalization, including antibiotics, surgery, and cardiovascular drugs.
Studies Performed: Electrocardiograms, CT scan.
Discharge medications:
Follow-up Arrangements:

Discharge Summary

Patient's Name and Medical Record Number:
Date of Admission:
Date of Discharge:
Admitting Diagnosis:
Discharge Diagnosis:
Attending or Ward Team Responsible for Patient:
Surgical Procedures, Diagnostic Tests, Invasive Procedures:
History, Physical Examination and Laboratory Data: Describe the course of the patient's disease up until the time that the patient came to the hospital, including pertinent physical exam and laboratory data.
Hospital Course: Describe the course of the patient's illness while in the hospital, including evaluation, treatment, medications, and outcome of treatment.
Discharged Condition: Describe improvement or deterioration in the patient's condition, and describe the present status of the patient.
Disposition: Note the situation to which the patient will be discharged (home), and indicate who will take care of the patient.
Discharge Medications: List medications and instructions for patient on taking the medications.
Discharge Instructions and Follow-up Care: Date of return for follow-up care at clinic; diet.
Problem List: List all active and past problems.
Copies: Send copies to attending, clinic, consultants.

Prescription Writing

- Patient's name:
- Date:
- Drug name and preparation (eg, tablets size): Lasix 40 mg
- Quantity to dispense: #40
- Frequency of administration: Sig: 1 po qAM
- Refills: None
- Signature

Procedure Note

A procedure note should be written in the chart after a procedure is performed. Procedure notes are brief operative notes.

Procedure Note

Date and time:
Procedure:
Indications:
Patient Consent: Document that the indications, risks and alternatives to the procedure were explained to the parents and patient. Note that the parents and patient were given the opportunity to ask questions and that the parents consented to the procedure in writing.
Lab tests: Relevant labs, such as the CBC and electrolytes.
Anesthesia: Local with 2% lidocaine.
Description of Procedure: Briefly describe the procedure, including sterile prep, anesthesia method, patient position, devices used, anatomic location of procedure, and outcome.
Complications and Estimated Blood Loss (EBL):
Disposition: Describe how the patient tolerated the procedure.
Specimens: Describe any specimens obtained and lab tests that were ordered.

Developmental Milestones

Age	Milestones
1 month	Raises head slightly when prone; alerts to sound; regards face, moves extremities equally.
2-3 months	Smiles, holds head up, coos, reaches for familiar objects, recognizes parent.
4-5 months	Rolls front to back and back to front; sits well when propped; laughs, orients to voice; enjoys looking around; grasps rattle, bears some weight on legs.
6 months	Sits unsupported; passes cube hand to hand; babbles; uses raking grasp; feeds self crackers.
8-9 months	Crawls, cruises; pulls to stand; pincer grasp; plays pat-a-cake; feeds self with bottle; sits without support; explores environment.

Age	Milestones
12 months	Walking, talking a few words; understands no; says mama/dada discriminantly; throws objects; imitates actions, marks with crayon, drinks from a cup.
15-18 months	Comes when called; scribbles; walks backward; uses 4-20 words; builds tower of 2 blocks.
24-30 months	Removes shoes; follows 2 step command; jumps with both feet; holds pencil, knows first and last name; knows pronouns. Parallel play; points to body parts, runs, spoon feeds self, copies parents.
3 years	Dresses and undresses; walks up and down steps; draws a circle; knows more than 250 words; takes turns; shares. Group play.
4 years	Hops, skips, catches ball; memorizes songs; plays cooperatively; knows colors; uses plurals.
5 years	Jumps over objects; prints first name; knows address and mother's name; follows game rules; draws three part man; hops on one foot.

12 Developmental Milestones

Cardiovascular Disorders

Chest Pain

Chief Complaint: Chest pain.

History of Present Illness: Duration of chest pain, location, character (squeezing, sharp, dull). Progression of pain, frequency, aggravating and relieving factors (inspiration, exertion, eating). Weight loss, fever, cough, dyspnea, vomiting, heartburn, abdominal pain. School function and attendance. Relationship of pain to activity (at rest, during sleep, during exercise). Does the pain interfere with the patient's daily activities? Have favorite sports or other activities continued?

Cardiac Testing: Results of prior evaluations, ECGs, echocardiograms.

Past Medical History: Exercise tolerance, diabetes, asthma, trauma.

Medications: Aspirin.

Family History: Heart disease, myocardial infarction, angina.

Social History: Significant life events, stresses, recent losses or separations. Elicit drugs, smoking.

Historical Findings for Chest Pain	
Acute pain? First time? Systemic symptoms? Duration of complaints? Exertional? Syncope? Palpitations? Cough? Localized? Reproducible? How? Associated symptoms?	Abdominal pain, limb pain, head-aches? Light-headedness, tetany, cramps, dizziness? Dermatomal distribution? Aggravated by rising from supine position? Poor school attendance? Stressful life events?

Physical Examination

General: Visible pain, apprehension, distress. Note whether the patient looks "ill" or well. Positions that accentuate or relieve the pain.

Vital Signs: Pulse (tachycardia), BP, respirations (tachypnea), temperature. Growth chart and percentiles.

Skin: Cold extremities, pallor.

Chest: Chest wall tenderness. Swelling, trauma, dermatomal lesions, breast development, gynecomastia, xiphoid process tenderness. Crackles, rhonchi, wheeze.

Heart: First and second heart sounds; third heart sound (S3), S4 gallop (more audible in the left lateral position), murmur.

Abdomen: Bowel sounds, tenderness, masses, hepatomegaly, splenomegaly.

Back: Vertebral column deformities, tenderness.

Extremities: Unequal or diminished pulses (aortic coarctation).

Laboratory Evaluation: Electrolyte, CBC, chest X-ray.

Differential Diagnosis of Chest Pain

Musculoskeletal Disorders	**Cardiovascular Disease**
Costochondritis	Pericarditis
Chest wall syndrome	Left ventricular outflow
Tietze syndrome	obstruction, aortic murmur
Xiphoid cartilage syndrome	Dysrhythmias
Stitch	**Pulmonary Disorders:** Pneumonia,
Precordial catch syndrome	pneumothorax, asthma
Slipping rib syndrome	**Gastrointestinal Disorders:**
Idiopathic Disorders: Psychogenic,	Esophagitis, gastroesophageal reflux,
hyperventilation	peptic ulcer disease
Breast Disorders: Gynecomastia,	**Vertebral/Radicular Disorders**
fibrocystic changes	Spinal stenosis
	Herniated disk
	Vertebral fracture

Dyspnea and Congestive Heart Failure

Chief Complaint: Shortness of breath.

History of Present Illness: Rate of onset of dyspnea (gradual, sudden), dyspnea on exertion, chest pain. Past episodes, aggravating or relieving factors, cough, fever, drug allergies. Difficulty keeping up with peers during play. Feeding difficulty, tachypnea or diaphoresis with feedings, diminished volume of feeding, prolonged feeding time. Poor weight gain.

Past Medical History: Hypertension, asthma, diabetes.

Medications: Bronchodilators, digoxin, furosemide.

Past Treatment or Testing: Cardiac testing, x-rays, ECGs.

Physical Examination

General Appearance: Respiratory distress, dyspnea, pallor. Note whether the patient looks "ill" or well.

Vital Signs: BP (supine and upright), pulse (tachycardia), temperature, respiratory rate (tachypnea), growth percentiles, growth deficiency.

HEENT: Jugular venous distention.

Chest: Intercostal retractions, dullness to percussion, stridor, wheezing, crackles, rhonchi.

Heart: Lateral displacement of point of maximal impulse, hyperdynamic precordium; irregular, rhythm; S3 gallop, S4, murmur.

Abdomen: Hepatomegaly, liver tenderness, splenomegaly.

Extremities: Cool extremities, edema, pulses, cyanosis, clubbing.

Laboratory Evaluation: O_2 saturation, chest x-ray (cardiomegaly, effusions, pulmonary edema).

Differential Diagnosis: Heart failure, foreign body aspiration, pneumonia, asthma, pneumothorax, hyperventilation.

Hypertension

Chief Complaint: High blood pressure.

History of Present Illness: Current blood pressure, age of onset of hypertension. Headaches, vomiting (increased intracranial pressure), dysuria, nocturia, enuresis, abdominal pain (renal disease). Growth delay, weight loss, fevers, diaphoresis, flushing, palpitations (pheochromocytoma).

Perinatal History: Neonatal course, umbilical artery/vein catheterization (renal artery stenosis).

Past Medical History: Lead exposure; increased appetite, hyperactivity, tremors, heat intolerance (hyperthyroidism).

Medications Associated with Hypertension: Oral contraceptives, corticosteroids, cocaine, amphetamines, nonsteroidal antiinflammatory drugs.

Family History: Hypertension, preeclampsia, renal disease, pheochromocytoma.

Social History: Tobacco, alcohol.

Physical Examination

General Appearance: Confusion, agitation (hypertensive encephalopathy).

Vital Signs: Tachycardia (hyperthyroidism), fever (connective tissue disorder). BP in all extremities, pulse, asymmetric, respiratory rate.

Skin: Pallor (renal disease), café au lait spots, hypopigmented lesions (Von Recklinghausen's disease, tuberous sclerosis), lymphedema (Turner's syndrome), rashes (connective tissue disease), striae, hirsutism (Cushing's syndrome), plethora (pheochromocytoma).

HEENT: Papilledema, thyromegaly (hyperthyroidism), moon faces (Cushing's syndrome); webbing of the neck (Turner's syndrome, aortic coarctation).

Chest: Crackles (pulmonary edema), wheeze, intercostal bruits (aortic coarctation); buffalo hump (Cushing's syndrome).

Heart: Delayed radial to femoral pulses (aortic coarctation). Laterally displaced apical impulse (ventricular hypertrophy), murmur.

Abdomen: Bruit below costal margin (renal artery stenosis); Masses (pheochromocytoma, neuroblastoma, Wilms' tumor). pulsating aortic mass (aortic aneurysm), enlarged kidney (polycystic kidney disease, hydronephrosis); costovertebral angle tenderness; truncal obesity (Cushing's syndrome).

Extremities: Edema (renal disease), joint swelling, joint tenderness (connective tissue disease). Tremor (hyperthyroidism, pheochromocytoma), femoral bruits.

Neurologic: Rapid return phase of deep tendon reflexes (hyperthyroidism).

Laboratory Evaluation: Potassium, BUN, creatinine, glucose, uric acid, CBC. UA with microscopic analysis (RBC casts, hematuria, proteinuria). 24 hour urine for metanephrine; plasma catecholamines (pheochromocytoma), lipid profile. Echocardiogram, ECG, renal ultrasound.

Chest X-ray: Cardiomegaly, indentation of aorta (coarctation), rib notching.

Differential Diagnosis of Hypertension

Renal

Chronic pyelonephritis
Chronic glomerulonephritis
Hydronephrosis
Congenital dysplastic kidney
Multicystic kidney
Solitary renal cyst
Vesicoureteral reflux nephropathy

Segmental hypoplasia
Ureteral obstruction
Renal tumors
Renal trauma
Systemic lupus erythematosus
(other connective tissue diseases)

Vascular

Coarctation of the aorta
Renal artery lesions
Umbilical artery catheterization with thrombus formation

Neurofibromatosis
Renal vein thrombosis
Vasculitis

Endocrine

Hyperthyroidism
Hyperparathyroidism
Congenital adrenal hyperplasia
Cushing syndrome
Hyperaldosteronism

Pheochromocytoma
Neuroblastoma, ganglioneuro-
blastoma, ganglioneuroma
Diabetic nephropathy
Liddle's syndrome

Central Nervous System

Intracranial mass
Hemorrhage

Brain injury
Quadriplegia

Essential Hypertension

Low renin
Normal renin

High renin

Pulmonary Disorders

Wheezing and Asthma

Chief Complaint: Wheezing.

History of Present Illness: Onset, duration and progression of wheezing; current and baseline peak flow rate; severity of attack compared to previous episodes; fever, frequency of hospitalizations; home nebulizer use; cough.

Aggravating factors: Exercise, cold air, viral or respiratory infections, exposure to dust mites, animal dander. Seasons that provoke symptoms; foreign body aspiration.

Past Medical History: Previous episodes, pneumonia, recurrent croup, allergic rhinitis, food allergies. Baseline arterial blood gas results; pulmonary function testing.

Perinatal History: Prematurity (bronchopulmonary dysplasia),

Family History: Asthma, allergies, hay fever, atopic dermatitis.

Physical Examination

General Appearance: Respiratory distress, anxiety, pallor. Note whether the patient looks well, ill, or somnolent.

Vital Signs: Peak expiratory flow rate (PEFR). Temperature, respiratory rate (tachypnea), depth of respirations, pulse (tachycardia), BP (widened pulse pressure), pulsus paradoxus (>15 mmHg is significant pulmonary compromise).

Skin: Flexural eczema, urticaria.

Nose: Nasal flaring, chronic rhinitis, nasal polyps.

Mouth: Pharyngeal erythema, perioral cyanosis, grunting.

Chest: Sternocleidomastoid muscle contractions, intracostal retractions, supraclavicular retractions, barrel chest. Expiratory wheeze, rhonchi, decreased breath sounds, prolonged expiratory phase.

Heart: Distant heart sounds, third heart sound (S3); increased intensity of pulmonic component of second heart sound (pulmonary hypertension).

Abdomen: Retractions, paradoxical abdominal wall motion (abdomen rises on inspiration), tenderness.

Extremities: Cyanosis, clubbing, edema.

Laboratory Evaluation: CBC, electrolytes. Pulmonary function tests, urinalysis.

ABG: Respiratory alkalosis, hypoxia.

Chest X-ray: Hyperinflation, flattening of diaphragms; small, elongated heart.

Differential Diagnosis of Wheezing	
Infant	**Older Child**
Vascular ring	Asthma
Tracheoesophageal fistula	Aspiration (reflux, foreign body)
Gastroesophageal reflux	Epiglottitis
Asthma	Laryngotracheobronchitis (croup)
Viral infection (bronchiolitis, upper respiratory tract infection)	Cystic fibrosis
	Hypersensitivity pneumonitis
Pertussis	Tuberculosis
Cystic fibrosis	Tumor
Bronchopulmonary dysplasia	Alpha$_1$-antitrypsin deficiency
Congenital heart disease	Vocal cord dysfunction

Stridor and Oropharyngeal Obstruction

Chief Complaint: Difficulty breathing.

History of Present Illness: Time of onset of stridor, respiratory distress. Fever, sore throat, headache, malaise. Voice changes (muffled voice), drooling. Hoarseness, exposure to infections. Trauma or previous surgery.

Increased stridor with stress; worsening in the supine position; improvement with the neck extended (congenital laryngomalacia). Cough, cyanosis, regurgitation, choking with feedings, drooling, foreign body. History of intubation (subglottic stenosis), hemangiomas.

Perinatal History: Abnormal position in utero, forceps delivery, shoulder dystocia. Respiratory distress or stridor at birth.

Historical Evaluation of Stridor and Oropharyngeal Obstruction	
Oropharyngeal Obstruction	**Stridor**
Fever, sore throat, headache	Gradual onset
Muffled voice	Acute onset, fever
Craniofacial anomalies	Worsens in supine position
Cutaneous abnormalities	Perinatal trauma
Neurologic symptoms	Method of delivery
	Present at birth
	Feeding difficulties
	Previous intubation

Physical Examination

General Appearance: Adequacy of oxygenation and ventilation, airway stability. Anxiety, restlessness, fatigue, obtundation. Grunting respirations, muffled voice, hoarseness, stridor.

Vital Signs: Respiratory rate, tachypnea, shallow breathing. Pulse oximetry. Tachycardia, fever. Growth percentiles.

Head: Congenital anomalies.

Skin: Perioral cyanosis, nail cyanosis, clubbing.
Nose: Nasal flaring.
Mouth: Bifid uvula, cleft palate. Symmetrical palate movement. Brisk gag reflex, tonsil symmetry. Tongue symmetry, movement in all directions, masses.
Neck: Masses, external fistulas, mid-line trachea.
Heart: Murmurs, abnormal pulses, asymmetric blood pressures.
Chest: Wall movement and symmetry, retractions, chest diameter, accessory muscle use (severe obstruction), hyperresonance, wheezes.
Abdomen: Retractions, paradoxical abdominal wall motion (abdomen rises on inspiration), tenderness.
Extremities: Cyanosis, clubbing, edema.

Physical Examination Findings in Stridor and Oropharyngeal Obstruction

Anxiety, fatigue, lethargy	Increased anteroposterior chest diameter
Cyanosis	Accessory muscle use
Tachypnea	Mouth-breathing
Hyperpnea	Grunting, nasal flaring
Shallow breaths	Muffled voice
Pulse oximeter <95 %	Hyponasal speech
Poor growth	Hypernasal speech
Clubbing	Low-pitched, fluttering sound
Heart murmur	Aphonia
Congenital head and neck anomalies	Quiet, moist stridor
Bifid uvula	Stridor
Enlarged tonsil(s)	Asymmetric wheezes
Neck mass	Neck extended
Asymmetric chest expansion	Opisthotonic posture
Retractions	Torticollis

Differential Diagnosis of Oropharyngeal Obstruction

Micrognathia	Retropharyngeal abscess
Pierre Robin syndrome	Parapharyngeal abscess
Treacher Collins syndrome	Hemangioma
Macroglossia	Lymphangioma
Down syndrome	Ranula
Beckwith-Wiedemann syndrome	Lymphoma
Lymphangioma	Lymphosarcoma
Hemangioma	Rhabdomyosarcoma
Lingual thyroid	Fibrosarcoma
Tonsillitis/hypertrophy: Bacterial, viral	Epidermoid carcinoma
Uvulitis	Adenoidal hypertrophy
Peritonsillar abscess	Palatal hypotonia
	Obesity

Differential Diagnosis of Stridor	
Neonatal	**Older Child**
Laryngomalacia Subglottic stenosis Webs Laryngeal cysts Tracheal stenosis Tracheomalacia Tracheal cartilage ring defect Laryngeal/tracheal ring calcification Vascular ring Pulmonary sling Innominate artery tracheal compression Vocal cord paralysis (Arnold-Chiari malformation, Dandy-Walker cyst, recurrent laryngeal nerve injury) Tumor Trauma (intubation, thermal injury, corrosive, gastric secretions)	Oropharyngeal infection (peritonsillar abscess, retropharyngeal abscess, tonsillitis) Viral infections (croup) Epiglottitis Bacterial tracheitis Aspirated/swallowed foreign body Tumor (hemangioma, lymphangioma)

Hoarseness

Chief Complaint: Hoarseness.

History of Present Illness: Age and time of onset, duration of symptoms, rate of onset, respiratory distress. Fever, hemangiomas, sore throat; prolonged loud crying or screaming (vocal chord polyps or nodules). Trauma or previous surgery; exposure to infections, exacerbating or relieving factors.

Perinatal History: Abnormal position in utero, shoulder dystocia, hyperextended neck during delivery (excessive neck traction). Respiratory distress or stridor at birth.

Past Medical History: Intubation (subglottic stenosis); prior episodes of croup, upper respiratory tract infections. Neurologic disorders (hydrocephalus, Arnold-Chiari malformation), trauma, previous surgery.

Physical Examination

General Appearance: Hoarseness, abnormal sounds/posture, muffled voice; hyponasal speech, hypernasal speech, quiet, moist stridor, inspiratory stridor, biphasic stridor; tachypnea.

Vital Signs: Respiratory rate (tachypnea), tachycardia, temperature. Delayed growth parameters.

Mouth: Tongue symmetry, movement in all directions, masses. Cleft lip, cleft palate, bifid uvula, enlarged tonsil(s). Mouth-breathing, grunting, nasal flaring;

Neck: Congenital anomalies; neck mass, masses or external fistulas, mid-line trachea.

Cardiac: Murmurs, asymmetric blood pressures.

Chest: Asymmetric chest expansion, retractions, increased anteroposterior chest diameter; accessory muscle use, abnormal vocal fremitus, wheezes, asymmetric wheezes; upright posture, neck extended, opisthotonic posture, torticollis.

Extremities: Cyanosis, clubbing.

Differential Diagnosis of Hoarseness	
Neonatal	**Older Child**
Laryngomalacia	Postnasal drip
Webs	Epiglottitis
Subglottic stenosis	Recurrent voice abuse (cord
Cystic lesions	polyps, nodules)
Excessive secretions (fistulas,	Sicca syndromes
gastroesophageal reflux)	Neoplasia (papilloma, heman-
Vascular tumors (hemangioma,	gioma)
lymphangioma)	Trauma (postsurgical, intubation)
Cri du chat syndrome	Gaucher disease,
Vocal cord paralysis	mucopolysaccharidosis
Vocal cord trauma	Williams syndrome, Cornelia de
Hypothyroidism, hypocalcemia,	Lange syndrome
Farber disease	Conversion reaction
Viral infection (laryngitis, croup)	

Infectious Diseases

Fever

Chief Complaint: Fever.

History of Present Illness: Degree of fever; time of onset, pattern of fever; cough, sputum, sore throat, headache, abdominal pain, ear pain, neck stiffness, dysuria; vomiting, rash, night sweats. Diarrhea, bone or joint pain, vaginal discharge.

Past Medical History: Ill contacts. Exposure to mononucleosis; exposure to tuberculosis or hepatitis; tuberculin skin testing; travel history, animal exposure; recent dental procedure.

Medications: Antibiotics, anticonvulsants.

Allergies: Drug allergies.

Family History: Familial Mediterranean fever, streptococcal disease, connective tissue disease.

Social History: Alcohol use, smoking.

Review of Systems: Breaks in the skin (insect bites or stings), weight loss, growth curve failure. Previous surgery or dental work. Heart murmur, AIDS risk factors.

Historical Findings in Fever of Unknown Origin

Skin breaks? Puncture or laceration.
Insect bites? Tick exposure, flies or mosquitoes.
Unusual or poorly prepared foods? Raw fish, unpasteurized milk.
Onset, periodicity, temperature curve, weight loss, school absence?
Localized pain?
Fever pattern?
Exposures or travel?
Pets? Kitten exposure, exposure to other animals.
Drugs? Any medication.

Review of systems? Rashes, joint complaints, cough, bowel movements.
Blood, urine, stool, and throat cultures?
Complete blood count? Inflammatory disorders usually lead to a rise in leukocyte count. Falling counts suggest a marrow process.
Screening laboratory procedures? Rise in sedimentation rate.
Tuberculin skin test with controls?

Physical Examination

General Appearance: Lethargy, toxic appearance. Note whether the patient looks "ill" or well.

Vital Signs: Temperature (fever curve), respiratory rate (tachypnea), pulse (tachycardia). Hypotension (sepsis), hypertension (neuroblastoma, pheochromocytoma). Growth and weight percentiles.

Skin: Rashes, nodules, skin breaks, bruises, pallor. Icterus, splinter hemorrhages; delayed capillary refill, petechia (septic emboli, meningococcemia), ecthyma gangrenosum (purpuric plaque of Pseudomonas). Pustules, cellulitis, furuncles, abscesses.

Lymph Nodes: Cervical, supraclavicular, axillary, inguinal adenopathy.
Eyes: Conjunctival erythema, retinal hemorrhages, papilledema.
Ears: Tympanic membrane inflammation, decreased mobility.
Mouth: Periodontitis, sinus tenderness; pharyngeal erythema, exudate.
Neck: Lymphadenopathy, neck rigidity.
Breast: Tenderness, masses, discharge.
Chest: Dullness to percussion, rhonchi, crackles.
Heart: Murmurs (rheumatic fever, endocarditis, myocarditis).
Abdomen: Masses, liver tenderness, hepatomegaly, splenomegaly; right lower quadrant tenderness (appendicitis). Costovertebral angle tenderness, suprapubic tenderness (urinary tract infection).
Extremities: Wounds; IV catheter tenderness (phlebitis) joint or bone tenderness (septic arthritis). Osler's nodes, Janeway's lesions (endocarditis). Clubbing, vertebral tenderness.
Rectal: Perianal skin tags, fissures, anal ulcers (Crohn disease), rectal flocculence, fissures, masses, occult blood.
Pelvic/Genitourinary: Cervical discharge, cervical motion tenderness, adnexal tenderness, adnexal masses, genital herpes lesions.

Laboratory Evaluation of Fever

Complete blood count, including leukocyte differential and platelet count	Serum lactate
	Cultures with antibiotic sensitivities
Electrolytes	Blood
Arterial blood gases	Urine
Blood urea nitrogen and creatinine	Wound
Urinalysis	Sputum, drains
INR, partial thromboplastin time, fibrinogen	Chest x-ray
	Computed tomography, magnetic resonance imaging, abdominal X-ray

Differential Diagnosis of Fever

Infectious Disease (50% of diagnoses)
Localized Infection
Respiratory tract
  Upper--rhinitis, pharyngitis, sinusitis
  Lower--pneumonia, bronchitis, bronchiectasis, foreign body
Urinary tract infection
Osteomyelitis
Meningitis, encephalitis
Abdominal abscess, appendicitis
Generalized Infection
Common--Epstein-Barr virus, enteric infection (Salmonella, Yersinia species), cat-scratch disease, tuberculosis, hepatitis, cytomegalovirus
Unusual--tularemia, brucellosis, leptospirosis, Q fever, Lyme disease, syphilis, toxoplasmosis

Collagen/Connective Tissue Disorders
Juvenile rheumatoid arthritis
Kawasaki syndrome
Systemic lupus
Rheumatic fever
Other: Vasculitis syndromes, Behçet's disease, mixed connective tissue disease

Neoplasia
Lymphoreticular malignancies
Sarcomas
Inflammatory Bowel Disease
Crohn disease

Periodic Fever
Recurrent viral infections
Cyclic neutropenia, familial Mediterranean fever (serositis, arthritis), "pharyngitis with aphthous stomatitis" (Marshall syndrome), Borrelia infection, familial dysautonomia
Pseudo-fever of Unknown Origin: Prolonged low-grade fevers without findings on examination, multiple vague complaints, normal laboratory tests

Cough and Pneumonia

Chief Complaint: Cough

History of Present Illness: Duration of cough, fever. Sputum color, quantity, consistency. Sore throat, rhinorrhea, headache, ear pain; vomiting, chest pain, hemoptysis. Travel history, exposure to tuberculosis, tuberculin testing. Timing of the cough, frequency of cough; cough characteristics. Dry, "brassy" cough (tracheal or large airway origins). Cough that is most notable when attention is drawn to it (psychogenic cough). Exposure to other persons with cough.

Past Medical History: Previous hospitalizations, prior radiographs. Diabetes, asthma, immunodeficiencies, chronic pulmonary disease.

Medications: Antibiotics

Immunizations: H influenzae, streptococcal immunization.

Allergies: Drug Allergies

Perinatal History: Respiratory distress syndrome, bronchopulmonary dysplasia, congenital pneumonias.

Psychosocial History: Daycare or school attendance, school absences, stressors within the family, tobacco smoke.

Family History: Atopy, asthma, cystic fibrosis, tuberculosis, recurrent infections.

Review of Systems: General state of health; growth and development; feeding history, conjunctivitis, choking, abnormal stools, neuromuscular weakness.

Physical Examination

General Appearance: Respiratory distress, cyanosis, dehydration. Note whether the patient looks "ill" well.

Vital Signs: Temperature (fever), respiratory rate (tachypnea), pulse (tachycardia), BP, height and weight percentiles.

Skin: Eczema, urticaria.

Lymph Nodes: Cervical, axillary, inguinal lymphadenopathy

Ears: Tympanic membrane erythema.

Nose: Nasal polyps.

Throat: Pharyngeal cobblestone follicles, pharyngeal erythema, masses, tonsillar enlargement.

Neck: Rigidity, masses, thyroid masses.

Chest: Chest wall deformities, asymmetry, unequal expansion. Increased vocal fremitus, dullness to percussion, wheezing, rhonchi, crackles; bronchial breath sounds with decreased intensity.

Heart: Tachypnea, gallops, murmurs (rheumatic fever, endocarditis, myocarditis).

Abdomen: Hepatomegaly, splenomegaly.

Extremities: Cyanosis, clubbing.

Neurologic: Decreased mental status, gag reflex, muscle tone and strength, swallowing coordination.

Laboratory Evaluation: CBC, electrolytes, BUN, creatinine; O_2 saturation, UA. WBC (>15,000 cells/dL). Sputum or deep tracheal aspirate for Gram's stain and culture. Tuberculin skin test (PPD), cultures and fluorescent antibody techniques for respiratory viruses.

Chest X-ray: Segmental consolidation, air bronchograms, atelectasis, pleural effusion.

Differential Diagnosis of Cough by Age		
Infant	Toddler/Young School-Age	Older School-Age/Adolescent
Infections	Viral infections	Asthma
Viral/bacterial infections	Sinusitis	Recurrent viral infections
Tuberculosis	Tuberculosis	Sinusitis
Gastroesophageal reflux	Gastroesophageal reflux	Tuberculosis
Anomalies	Inhaled foreign body	Mycoplasma
Vascular ring	Desquamative interstitial pneumonitis	Gastroesophageal reflux
Innominate artery compression	Lymphocytic interstitial pneumonitis	Psychogenic cough
Tracheoesophageal fistula	Asthma	Cystic fibrosis
Pulmonary sequestration	Cough-variant asthma	Bronchiectasis
Subglottic stenosis	Pollutants (cigarette smoke)	Immunodeficiency
Interstitial pneumonia	Suppurative lung disease	
Desquamative interstitial pneumonia	Cystic fibrosis	
Lymphocytic interstitial pneumonitis	Bronchiectasis	
Asthma	Right middle lobe syndrome	
Cystic fibrosis	Ciliary dyskinesia syndromes	
Ciliary dyskinesia syndromes		
Immunodeficiency		

Tuberculosis

Chief Complaint: Cough and fever.

History of Present Illness: Tuberculin skin test (PPD) results; duration of cough, sputum, fever, headache. Stiff neck, bone pain, joint pain. Prior treatment for tuberculosis. Exposure to tuberculosis. Chest roentgenogram results. Sputum color, quantity, consistency, hemoptysis. Urban, low-income population, homeless.

Travel History: Travel to South America, Southeast Asia, India.

Past Medical History: Previous pneumonia, previous hospitalizations, prior radiographs, AIDS risk factors. Diabetes, asthma, steroids, immunodeficiencies, chronic pulmonary disease.

Medications: Antihistamines.

Allergies: Drug allergies.

Family History: Source case drug resistance. Tuberculosis, recurrent infections, chronic lung disease.

Review of Systems: General state of health; growth and development; feeding history, abnormal stools, neuromuscular weakness.

Social History: Daycare or school attendance.

Physical Examination

General Appearance: Respiratory distress. Note whether the patient looks "ill" or well.

Vital Signs: Temperature (fever), respiratory rate (tachypnea), pulse (tachycardia), BP, growth percentiles.

Skin: Rashes, cyanosis, urticaria.

Lymph Nodes: Lymphadenopathy (cervical, supraclavicular, axillary, inguinal).

HEENT: Tympanic membrane erythema, neck stiffness.

Chest: Increased vocal fremitus. Increased percussion resonance, rhonchi, crackles, bronchial breath sounds with decreased intensity.

Cardiac: Distant heart sounds, murmur, rub.

Abdomen: Masses, tenderness, hepatomegaly, splenomegaly.

Extremities: Clubbing, edema.

Neurologic: Mental status, muscle tone and strength.

Laboratory Evaluation: CBC, electrolytes, BUN, creatinine; O_2 saturation, liver function tests; UA, early morning gastric aspirate to obtain swallowed sputum for acid-fast bacilli stain and culture. Histological examination of lymph nodes, pleura, liver, bone marrow biopsies.

Chest X-ray: Segmental consolidation, hilar node enlargement, segmental atelectasis.

Differential Diagnosis: Atypical mycobacteria infection, active pulmonary tuberculosis, latent tuberculosis.

Otitis Media

Chief Complaint: Ear pain.

History of Present Illness: Ear pain, fever, irritability. Degree of fever; time of onset; cough, sore throat, headache, neck stiffness, diarrhea.

Past Medical History: Previous episodes of otitis media, pneumonia, asthma, diabetes, immunosuppression, steroid use.

Allergies: Antibiotics.
Family History: Recurrent ear infections.

Physical Examination
Ears: Bulging, opacified, erythematous tympanic membrane; poor visualization of landmarks, absent light reflex , retraction, decreased mobility with insufflation of air.
Nose: Nasal discharge, erythema.
Throat: Pharyngeal erythema, exudate.
Chest: Breath sounds.
Heart: Rate and rhythm, murmurs.
Abdomen: Tenderness, hepatomegaly.
Laboratory Evaluation: CBC, electrolytes, tympanocentesis.
Differential Diagnosis: Acute otitis media, mastoiditis, otitis externa, otitis media with effusion, cholesteatoma, tympanosclerosis, cholesteatoma.

Pharyngitis

Chief Complaint: Sore throat.
History of Present Illness: Sore throat, fever, cough, irritability, ear pain. Nasal discharge, headache, abdominal pain; prior streptococcal pharyngitis, past streptococcal pharyngitis, scarlet fever, rheumatic fever.
Past Medical History: Previous episodes of otitis media, pneumonia, asthma, diabetes, immunosuppression.
Allergies: Antibiotics.
Family History: Streptococcal throat infections.

Physical Examination
General Appearance: Note whether the patient appears well or toxic.
Vital Signs: Temperature (fever), pulse, blood pressure, respiratory rate.
Skin: Rash ("sandpaper" feel, scarlet fever).
Lymph Nodes: Tender cervical adenopathy.
Ears: Tympanic membrane erythema, bulging.
Nose: Mucosal erythema.
Throat: Erythema, vesicles, ulcers, soft palate petechiae. Tonsillar exudate.
Mouth: Foul breath.
Abdomen: Tenderness (mesenteric adenitis), hepatomegaly, splenomegaly.

Clinical Manifestations of Pharyngitis

	Group A streptococcus	Viral (other than EBV)	Epstein-Barr virus
Age	Generally 3 years or older	Any age	Over 5 yrs (especially late school age/adolescent)
Season	Fall to spring	Any	Any
Clinical	Tender cervical adenopathy, foul breath, tonsillar exudates, soft palate petechiae, abdominal pain (mesenteric adenitis), headache, rash ("sandpaper" feel, scarlet fever), no rhinorrhea, no cough, conjunctivitis (ie, no URI symptoms)	Papular-vesicular lesions or tonsillar ulcers (eg, herpangina, Coxsackie A), URI symptoms. Rash, often papulosquamous.	Indolent onset, tonsillar exudates, lymphadenopathy, fatigue, hepatosplenomegaly, atypical lymphocytes in peripheral smear. Rash with penicillin. Illness lasts more than 7-10 days (GABHS infection resolves within 7 days).

Laboratory Evaluation: Rapid antigen detection test, throat culture.
Differential Diagnosis of Pharyngitis: Viruses (influenza, adenovirus. Epstein-Barr virus), groups C and G streptococci, Corynebacterium diphtheriae (gray exudate in the pharynx), Chlamydia.

Peritonsillar, Retropharyngeal or Parapharyngeal Abscess

Chief Complaint: Throat pain.
History of Present Illness: Recent tonsillopharyngitis or URI. Stridor, dysphagia, drooling.
Past Medical History: Previous peritonsillar abscesses, pharyngitis, otitis media, pneumonia, asthma, diabetes, immunosuppression.
Medications: Immunosuppressants.
Allergies: Antibiotics.
Family History: Streptococcal pharyngitis.

Physical Examination
General Appearance: Severe throat pain and dysphagia. Ill appearance.
Throat: Trismus, "hot potato voice," uvula pointing toward unaffected side (peritonsillar abscess). Stridor, drooling, anterior pharyngeal wall displacement (retropharyngeal abscess).
Lymph Nodes: Cervical lymphadenopathy.
Chest: Breath sounds, rhonchi.
Heart: Murmurs, rubs.
Abdomen: Tenderness, hepatomegaly, splenomegaly.
Laboratory Evaluation: Cultures of surgical drainage. Lateral neck X ray.

Epiglottitis

Chief Complaint: Sore throat.
History of Present Illness: 3 to 7 years of age and an abrupt onset of high fever, severe sore throat, dysphagia, drooling. Refusal to swallow, drooling; quiet, hoarse voice.
Past Medical History: Immunosuppression.
Medications: Immunosuppressants.
Vaccinations: Haemophilus influenza immunization.

Physical Examination
General Appearance: Inspiratory stridor, "toxic" appearance. Respiratory distress (sitting in tripod posture with neck extended), apprehension.
Chest: Stridor, decreased breath sounds.
Heart: Murmurs.
Abdomen: Tenderness, splenomegaly.
Extremities: Cyanosis.
Laboratory Evaluation: Lateral neck x-rays

Differential Diagnosis of Epiglottitis		
Epiglottitis	**Viral Laryngo-tracheitis**	**Bacterial Tracheitis**
High fever, dysphagia, drooling, "toxic" appearance, refusal to speak	Low-grade fever, coryza. barking cough, hoarse voice	Improving croup that worsens; high fever, stridor, anterior neck tenderness: no drooling

Croup (Viral Laryngotracheobronchitis)

Chief Complaint: Cough.
History of Present Illness: Mild upper respiratory symptoms, followed by sudden onset of a barking cough and hoarseness, often at night.
Past Medical History: Immunosuppression.
Past Medical History: Prematurity, respiratory distress syndrome, bronchopulmonary dysplasia.
Medications: Antibiotics.
Vaccinations: Haemophilus influenza immunization.

Physical Examination
General Appearance: Low-grade fever, non-toxic appearance. Comfortable at rest, barky, seal-like cough. Restlessness, altered mental status.
Vital Signs: Respirations (tachypnea), blood pressure, pulse (tachycardia), temperature (low-grade fever).
Skin: Pallor, cyanosis.
Chest: Inspiratory stridor, tachypnea, retractions, diminished breath sounds.
Abdomen: Retractions, paradoxical abdominal wall motion (abdomen rises on inspiration), tenderness.
Laboratory Evaluation: Anteroposterior neck radiographs: subglottic narrowing, ("steeple sign"); pulse oximetry.
Differential Diagnosis: Epiglottitis, acute croup, foreign body aspiration, anaphylaxis; spasmodic croup (recurrent allergic upper airway spasm).

Bronchiolitis

Chief Complaint: Wheezing.
History of Present Illness: Duration of wheezing, cough, mild fever, nasal discharge, congestion. Cold weather months. Oxygen saturation.
Past Medical History: Chronic pulmonary disease (ie, prematurity, bronchopulmonary dysplasia), heart disease, immunocompromise.
Medications: Bronchodilators.
Allergies: Aspirin, food allergies.
Family History: Asthma, hayfever, eczema.
Social History: Exposure to passive cigarette smoke.

Physical Examination

General Appearance: Comfortable appearing, non-toxic.

Vital Signs: Temperature (low-grade fever), respirations, pulse, blood pressure.

Ears: Tympanic membrane erythema.

Nose: Rhinorrhea

Mouth: Flaring of the nostrils.

Chest: Chest wall retractions, wheezing, fine crackles on inspiration, diminished air exchange.

Heart: Murmurs.

Abdomen: Paradoxical abdominal wall motion with respiration (ie, abdomen collapses with each inspiration).

Laboratory Evaluation: CBC, electrolytes, pulse oximetry. Nasopharyngeal washings for RSV antigen.

Chest X-ray: Hyperinflation, flattened diaphragms, patchy atelectasis.

Differential Diagnosis: Foreign body aspiration, asthma, pneumonia, congestive heart failure, aspiration syndromes (gastroesophageal reflux).

Meningitis

Chief Complaint: Fever and lethargy.

History of Present Illness: Duration and degree of fever; headache, neck stiffness, cough; lethargy, irritability (high-pitched cry), vomiting, anorexia, rash.

Past Medical History: Pneumonia, otitis media, endocarditis. Diabetes, sickle cell disease; recent upper respiratory infections. Travel history.

Perinatal History: Prematurity, respiratory distress.

Medications: Antibiotics.

Social History: Home situation.

Family History: Exposure to H influenza or neisseria meningitis.

Physical Examination

General Appearance: Level of consciousness; obtundation, labored respirations. Note whether the patient looks "ill," well, or malnourished.

Vital Signs: Temperature (fever), pulse (tachycardia), respiratory rate (tachypnea), BP (hypotension).

Skin: Capillary refill, rashes, petechia, purpura (meningococcemia).

Head: Bulging or sunken fontanelle.

Eyes: Extraocular movements, papilledema, pupil reactivity, icterus.

Neck: Nuchal rigidity. Brudzinski's sign (neck flexion causes hip flexion); Kernig's sign (flexing hip and extending knee elicits resistance).

Chest: Rhonchi, crackles, wheeze.

Heart: Rate of rhythm, murmurs.

Extremities: Splinter hemorrhages (endocarditis).

Neurologic: Altered mental status, weakness, sensory deficits.

Laboratory Evaluation:

CSF Tube 1 - Gram stain, culture and sensitivity, bacterial antigen screen (1-2 mL).

CSF Tube 2 - Glucose, protein (1-2 mL).

CSF Tube 3 - Cell count and differential (1-2 mL).

Electrolytes, BUN, creatinine. CBC with differential, blood cultures, smears and cultures from purpuric lesions: cultures of stool, urine, joint fluid, abscess; purified protein derivative (PPD).

Cerebral Spinal Fluid Analysis				
Disease	Color	Protein	Cells	Glucose
Normal CSF Fluid	Clear	<50 mg/100 mL	<5 lymphs/mm'	>40 mg/100 mL, ½-2/3 of blood glucose level
Bacterial meningitis or tuberculous meningitis	Cloudy	Elevated 50-1500	>100 WBC/mm' predominantly neutrophils. Bacteria present on Gram's stain.	Low, <½ of blood glucose
Tuberculous, fungal, partially treated bacterial, syphilitic meningitis, meningeal metastases	Clear opalescent	Elevated usually <500	10-500 WBC with predominant lymphs	20-40, low
Viral meningitis, partially treated bacterial meningitis, encephalitis, toxoplasmosis	Clear opalescent	Slightly elevated or normal	10-500 WBC with predominant lymphs	Normal to low

Urinary Tract Infection

Chief Complaint: Pain with urination.

History of Present Illness: Dysuria, frequency (voiding repeatedly of small amounts), malodorous urine, incontinence; suprapubic pain, low-back pain, fever, chills (pyelonephritis), vomiting, irritability; constipation. Urine culture results (suprapubic aspiration or urethral catheterization).

Past Medical History: Urinary infections.

Signs and Symptoms of UTIs in Different Age Groups	
Age	Signs/Symptoms
Neonate/infant	Hypothermia, hyperthermia, failure to thrive. vomiting, diarrhea, sepsis, irritability, lethargy, jaundice, malodorous urine

Age	Signs/Symptoms
Toddler	Abdominal pain, vomiting, diarrhea, constipation, abnormal voiding pattern, malodorous urine, fever, poor growth
School age	Dysuria, frequency, urgency, abdominal pain, incontinence or secondary enuresis, constipation, malodorous urine, fever
Adolescent	Dysuria, frequency, urgency, abdominal pain, malodorous urine, fever

Physical Examination
General Appearance: Dehydration, septic appearance. Note whether the patient looks toxic or well.
Vital Signs: Temperature (high fever [>38°C] pyelonephritis), respiratory rate, pulse, BP.
Chest: Breath sounds.
Heart: Rhythm, murmurs.
Abdomen: Suprapubic tenderness, costovertebral angle tenderness (pyelonephritis), renal mass, nephromegaly. Lower abdominal mass (distended bladder), stool in colon.
Pelvic/Genitourinary: Circumcision, hypospadia, phimosis, foreskin; vaginal discharge.
Laboratory Evaluation: UA with micro, urine Gram stain, urine C&S. CBC with differential, electrolytes. Ultrasound, voiding cystourethrogram, renal nuclear scan.
Differential Diagnosis: Cystitis, pyelonephritis, vulvovaginitis, gonococcal or chlamydia urethritis, herpes infection, cervicitis, appendicitis, pelvic inflammatory disease.

Differential Diagnosis of Urinary Tract Symptoms

Urinary tract infection	Emotional disturbances
Urethritis	Vulvovaginitis
Urethral irritation by soaps, detergents, bubble bath	Trauma (sexual abuse)
Vaginal foreign bodies	Pinworms

Lymphadenopathy and Lymphadenitis

Chief Complaint: Swollen lymph nodes.
History of Present Illness: Duration of generalized or regional adenopathy. Fever, pattern, spiking fevers, relapsing fever, rash, arthralgias. Sore throat, nasal discharge, cough, travel history. Animal exposure (cat scratch, kittens).

Localized trauma or skin infection, exposure to tuberculosis, blood product exposure. Conjunctivitis, recurrent infections.

Past Medical History: Developmental delay, growth failure.

Social History: Intravenous drug use, high-risk sexual behavior.

Medications: Phenytoin.

Review of Systems: Weight loss, night sweats, bone pain. Pallor, easy bruising.

Historical Evaluation of Lymphadenopathy	
Generalized or regional adenopathy	Animal exposure
Fever	Blood product exposure
Rash	Arthralgia/arthritis
Exposure to infection	Delayed growth/development
Travel	Weight loss, night sweats
	Lesions at birth

Physical Examination

General Appearance: Dehydration, septic appearance. Note whether the patient looks toxic or well.

Vital Signs: Temperature (fever), pulse (tachycardia), blood pressure, wide pulse pressure (hyperthyroidism). Growth percentiles.

Lymph Nodes: Generalized or regional adenopathy. Location, size of enlarged lymph nodes; discreteness, mobility, consistency, tenderness, fluctuation. Supraclavicular or posterior triangle lymphadenopathy.

Skin: Lesion in the area(s) drained by affected lymph nodes. Sandpaper rash (scarlet fever), punctums, pustules, splinter hemorrhages (endocarditis), exanthems or enanthems, malar rash (systemic lupus erythematosus).

Eyes: Conjunctivitis, uveitis.

Chest: Breath sounds, wheeze, crackles.

Heart: Rhythm, murmurs.

Abdomen: Tenderness, masses, hepatomegaly splenomegaly.

Extremities: Joint swelling, joint tenderness, extremity lesions, nasopharyngeal masses.

Physical Examination Findings in Lymphadenopathy	
Generalized or regional adenopathy	Hepatosplenomegaly
Growth failure	Skin pustule/puncture
Fever	Conjunctivitis/uveitis
Tachycardia, wide pulse pressure, brisk reflexes	Midline neck mass that retracts with tongue protrusion
Rash/exanthem	Mass in posterior triangle
	Supraclavicular mass

Differential Diagnosis of Adenopathy Based on Location

Location of Node(s)	Etiology of Infection or Process
Posterior auricular, posterior/ suboccipital, occipital	Measles, scalp infections (eg, tinea capitis)
Submandibular, anterior cervical	Oropharyngeal or facial infections (unilateral, "cold" submandibular nodes without infection indicates atypical mycobacteria)
Preauricular	Sinusitis, tularemia
Posterior cervical	Adjacent skin infection
Bilateral cervical of marked degree	Kawasaki's disease, mononucleosis, toxoplasmosis, secondary syphilis
Supraclavicular or scalene, lower cervical	Infiltrative process (malignancy)
Axillary	Cat scratch disease, sporotrichosis
Generalized adenopathy, including axillary, epitrochlear, inguinal	Generalized infection (mononucleosis, hepatitis), immunodeficiency (HIV), sarcoidosis
Recurrent episodes of adenitis	Chronic granulomatous disease, immunodeficiency

Differential Diagnosis of Generalized Lymphadenopathy

Systemic Infections

Bacterial infections
Scarlet fever
Viral exanthems (eg, rubella or rubeola)
Epstein-Barr virus
Cytomegalovirus
Hepatitis virus
Cat-scratch disease
Mycoplasma organisms
Bacterial endocarditis

Tuberculosis
Syphilis
Toxoplasma organisms
Brucella organisms
Histoplasmosis
Coccidioidomycosis
Typhoid fever
Malaria
Chronic granulomatous disease
HIV infection

Immune-Mediated Inflammatory   Disorders

Systemic lupus erythematosus
Juvenile rheumatoid arthritis
Serum sickness

Kawasaki syndrome
Hyper IgD syndrome
Hyper IgE syndrome

Storage Diseases	
Gaucher disease Niemann-Pick disease	Tangier disease
Malignancies	
Leukemia Lymphoma Neuroblastoma	Histiocytosis X X-linked lymphoproliferative syndrome
Metabolic Disorders	
Hyperthyroidism	Adrenal insufficiency
Miscellaneous	
Drug reactions (phenytoin, allopurinol) Hemolytic anemias Immunoblastic lymphadenopathy	Sarcoidosis Sinus histiocytosis

Laboratory Evaluation: Throat culture, EBV, CMV, toxoplasmosis titers, CBC and differential, ESR, PPD. Blood cultures, chest X ray, VDRL. Needle aspiration of the node, after saline infusion, for Gram's stain and acid-fast stains, and culture for aerobes, anaerobes, and mycobacteria. Cat scratch bacillus (Bartonella henselae) titer.

Differential Diagnosis of Cervical Lymphadenopathy	

Viral upper respiratory tract infection
    (EBV or CMV infection)
Suppurative infections (staphylococcal,
    streptococcal)
Cold inflammation
Cat-scratch disease
Atypical mycobacterial adenitis
Toxoplasmosis
	Systemic disorders
	    Kawasaki syndrome
	    Kikuchi disease
	    Hyper IgD syndrome
	    Hyper IgE syndrome
	    Sinus histiocytosis
	    Sarcoidosis
	    Drugs

Cellulitis

Chief Complaint: Red skin lesion.
History of Present Illness: Warm, red, painful, indurated lesion. Fever, chills, headache; diarrhea, localized pain, night sweats. Insect bite or sting; joint pain.
Past Medical History: Cirrhosis, diabetes, heart murmur, recent surgery; AIDS risk factors.
Allergies: Drug allergies.
Review of Systems: Animal exposure (pets), travel history, drug therapy.
Family History: Diabetes, cancer.
Social History: Home situation.

Physical Examination
General Appearance: Note whether the patient looks "ill" or well.
Vital Signs: Temperature (fever curve), respiratory rate (tachypnea), pulse (tachycardia), BP (hypotension).
Skin: Warm, erythematous, tender, indurated lesion. Poorly demarcated erythema with flat borders. Bullae, skin breaks, petechia, ecthyma gangrenosum (purpuric of Pseudomonas), pustules, abscesses.
Lymph Nodes: Adenopathy localized or generalized lymphadenopathy.
HEENT: Conjunctival erythema, periodontitis, tympanic membrane inflammation, neck rigidity.
Chest: Rhonchi, crackles, dullness to percussion (pneumonia).
Heart: Murmurs (endocarditis).
Abdomen: Liver tenderness, hepatomegaly, splenomegaly. Costovertebral angle tenderness, suprapubic tenderness.
Extremities: Wounds, joint or bone tenderness (septic arthritis).
Laboratory Evaluation: CBC, ESR, blood cultures x 2, electrolytes, glucose, BUN, creatinine, UA, urine Gram stain, C&S; skin lesion cultures. Needle aspiration of border for Gram's stain and culture. Antigen detection studies.
Differential Diagnosis: Cellulitis, erysipelas, dermatitis, dermatophytosis.

Infective Endocarditis

Chief Complaint: Fever
History of Present Illness: Chronic fever, murmur, malaise, anorexia, weight loss, arthralgias, abdominal pain. Recent gastrointestinal procedure, urinary procedure, dental procedure. valvular disease, rheumatic fever, seizures, stroke.
Past Medical History: Congenital heart disease.

Physical Examination
General Appearance: Note whether the patient looks toxic or well.
Vital Signs: Blood pressure (hypotension), pulse (tachycardia), temperature (fever), respirations (tachypnea).
Eyes: Roth spots (white retinal patches with surrounding hemorrhage)
Chest: Crackles, rhonchi.
Heart: Regurgitant murmurs.
Skin: Petechiae, Janeway lesions, Osler's nodes, splinter hemorrhages.
Extremities: Edema, clubbing.
Abdomen: Hepatomegaly, splenomegaly, tenderness.
Neurologic: Weakness, sensory deficits.
Laboratory Studies: CBC (leukocytosis with left shift), ESR, CXR, ECG, blood cultures, urinalysis and culture, BUN/creatinine, cultures of intravenous lines and catheter tips; echocardiography.
Differential Diagnosis: Infective endocarditis, rheumatic fever, systemic infection, tuberculosis, urinary tract infection.

Septic Arthritis

Chief Complaint: Joint pain.

History of Present Illness: Joint pain and warmth, redness, swelling, decreased range of motion. Acute onset of fever, limp, or refusal to walk. Penetrating injuries or lacerations. Preexisting joint disease (eg, rheumatoid arthritis), prosthetic joint; sexually transmitted disease exposure.

Past Medical History: H. influenzae immunization, sickle cell anemia, M. tuberculosis exposure.

Physical Examination

General Appearance: Note whether the patient looks toxic or well.

Vital Signs: Temperature (fever), blood pressure (hypotension), pulse (tachycardia), respirations.

Skin: Erythema, skin puncture. Vesicular rash, petechia.

HEENT: Neck rigidity.

Chest: Crackles, rhonchi.

Heart: Murmurs, friction rub.

Abdomen: Tenderness, hepatomegaly, splenomegaly.

Extremities: Erythema, limitation in joint range of motion, joint tenderness, swelling. Refusal to change position.

Laboratory Evaluation: X-rays of joint (joint space distention, periosteal reaction), CT or MRI. Arthrocentesis for cell count, Gram's stain, glucose, mucin clot, cultures. Bone-joint scans (gallium, technetium). Blood cultures. Culture of cervix and urethra on Thayer-Martin media for gonorrhea. Lyme titer, anti-streptolysin-O titer.

Synovial Fluid Findings in Various Types of Arthritis			
	WBC Count/mm	% PMN	Joint Fluid:Blood Glucose Ratio
Septic arthritis	>50,000	.90	Decreased
Juvenile rheumatoid arthritis	<15,000-20,000	60	Normal to decreased
Lyme arthritis	15,000-100,000	50+	Normal

Differential Diagnosis: Septic arthritis, Lyme disease, juvenile rheumatoid arthritis, systemic lupus erythematosus, acute rheumatic fever, inflammatory bowel disease, leukemia (bone pain), synovitis, trauma, cellulitis.

Osteomyelitis

Chief Complaint: Leg pain.

History of Present Illness: Extremity pain, degree of fever, duration of fever, limitation of extremity use; refusal to use the extremity or bear weight. Hip pain, abdominal pain, penetrating trauma, dog or cat bite (Pasteurella multocida), human bites, immunocompromise, tuberculosis.

Past Medical History: Diabetes mellitus, sickle cell disease; surgery, prosthetic devices.
Medications: Immunosuppressants.
Social History: Intravenous drug abuse.

Physical Examination
General Appearance: Note whether the patient looks septic or well.
Vital Signs: Blood pressure (hypotension), pulse (tachycardia), temperature (fever), respirations (tachypnea).
Skin: Petechiae, cellulitis, rash.
Chest: Crackles, rhonchi.
Heart: Regurgitant murmurs.
Extremities: Point tenderness, swelling, warmth, erythema. Tenderness of femur, tibia, humerus.
Back: Tenderness over spinus processes.
Abdomen: Tenderness, rectal mass.
Feet: Puncture wounds.
Laboratory Evaluation: CBC (elevated WBC), ESR (>50), blood culture; X-rays (soft tissue edema), CT or MRI. Technetium bone scan.
Differential Diagnosis: Cellulitis, skeletal or blood neoplasia (Ewing's sarcoma, leukemia), bone infarction (hemoglobinopathy), hemophilia with bleeding, thrombophlebitis, child abuse/trauma, synovitis.

Gastrointestinal Disorders

Acute Abdominal Pain and the Acute Abdomen

Chief Complaint: Abdominal pain.
History of Present Illness: Duration of pain, location of pain; characteristics of pain (diffuse, burning, crampy, sharp, dull); constant or intermittent; frequency. Effect of eating, defecation, urination, movement. Characteristics of last bowel movement. Relation to last menstrual period.
Relationship to meals. What does the patient do when the pain occurs? Fever, chills, nausea, vomiting (bilious, undigested food, blood, sore throat, constipation, diarrhea, hematochezia, melena, anorexia, weight loss.
Past Medical History: Diabetes, asthma, prematurity, surgery. Endoscopies, X-rays.
Medications: Aspirin, NSAIDs, narcotics, anticholinergics, laxatives.
Family History. Abdominal pain in family members, peptic ulcer disease, irritable bowel syndrome.
Social History: Recent travel, change in food consumption, drugs or alcohol.
Review of Systems: Growth delay, weight gain, emesis, bloating, distension. Headache, fatigue, weakness, stress- or tension-related symptoms.

Physical Examination
General Appearance: Degree of distress, body positioning to relieve pain, nutritional status. Signs of dehydration, septic appearance.
Vitals: Temperature (fever), pulse (tachycardia), BP (hypertension, hypotension), respiratory rate and pattern (tachypnea).
Skin: Jaundice, petechia, pallor, rashes.
HEENT: Pale conjunctiva, pharyngeal erythema, pus, flat neck veins.
Lymph Nodes: Cervical axillary, periumbilical, inguinal lymphadenopathy, Virchow node (supraclavicular mass).
Abdomen
  Inspection: Distention, visible peristalsis (small bowel obstruction).
  Auscultation: Absent bowel sounds (late obstruction), high-pitched rushes (early obstruction), bruits.
  Palpation: Masses, hepatomegaly, liver texture (smooth, coarse), splenomegaly. Bimanual palpation of flank, nephromegaly. Rebound tenderness, hernias, (inguinal, femoral, umbilical); costovertebral angle tenderness. Retained fecal material, distended bladder (obstructive uropathy).
    McBurney's Point Tenderness: Located two-thirds of the way between umbilicus and anterior superior iliac spine (appendicitis).
    Iliopsoas Sign: Elevation of legs against examiner's hand causes pain, retrocecal appendicitis. Obturator sign: Flexion of right thigh and external rotation of thigh causes pain in pelvic appendicitis.
    Rovsing's Sign: Manual pressure and release at left lower quadrant causes referred pain at McBurney's point (appendicitis).
  Percussion: Liver and spleen span, tympany.
Rectal Examination: Impacted stool, masses, tenderness; gross or occult blood.
Perianal Examination: Fissures, fistulas, hemorrhoids, skin tags, soiling (fecal

or urinary incontinence).

Male Genital Examination: Hernias, undescended testes, hypospadias.

Female Genital Examination: Urethra, distal vagina, trauma; imperforate hymen. Pelvic examination in pubertal girls. Cervical discharge, adnexal tenderness, masses, cervical motion tenderness.

Extremities: Edema, digital clubbing.

Neurologic: Observation of the patient moving on and off of the examination table. Gait.

Laboratory Evaluation: CBC, electrolytes, liver function tests, amylase, lipase, UA, pregnancy test.

Chest X-ray: Free air under diaphragm, infiltrates.

Acute Abdomen X-ray Series: Flank stripe, subdiaphragmatic free air, distended loops of bowel, sentinel loop, air fluid levels, calcifications, fecaliths.

Differential Diagnosis of Acute Abdominal Pain

Generalized Pain: Intestinal obstruction, diabetic ketoacidosis, constipation, malrotation of the bowel, volvulus, sickle crisis, acute porphyria, musculoskeletal trauma, psychogenic pain.

Epigastrium: Gastroesophageal reflux, intestinal obstruction, gastroenteritis, gastritis, peptic ulcer disease, esophagitis, pancreatitis, perforated viscus.

Right Lower Quadrant: Appendicitis, intussusception, salpingitis, endometritis, endometriosis, ectopic pregnancy, hemorrhage or rupture of ovarian cyst, testicular torsion.

Right Upper Quadrant: Appendicitis, cholecystitis, hepatitis, gastritis, gonococcal perihepatitis (Fitz-Hugh-Curtis syndrome), pneumonia.

Left Upper Quadrant: Gastroesophageal reflux, peptic ulcer, gastritis, pneumonia, pancreatitis, volvulus, intussusception, sickle crisis.

Left Lower Quadrant: Volvulus, intussusception, mesenteric lymphadenitis, intestinal obstruction, sickle crisis, colitis, strangulated hernia, testicular torsion, psychogenic pain, inflammatory bowel disease, gastroenteritis, pyelonephritis, salpingitis, ovarian cyst, ectopic pregnancy, endometriosis.

Hypogastric/Pelvic: Cystitis, urolithiasis, appendicitis, pelvic inflammatory disease, ectopic pregnancy, strangulated hernia, endometriosis, ovarian cyst torsion, bladder distension.

Recurrent Abdominal Pain

Chief Complaint: Abdominal pain.

History of Present Illness: Quality of pain (burning, crampy, sharp, dull); location (diffuse or localized). Duration of pain, change in frequency; constant or intermittent.

Effect of eating, vomiting, defecation, urination, inspiration, movement and position. Characteristics of bowel movements. Relation to last menstrual period. Vomiting (bilious, undigested food, blood), constipation, diarrhea, hematochezia, melena; dysuria, hematuria, anorexia, weight loss. Relationship to meals; triggers and relievers of the pain (antacids). Relationship to the menstrual cycle.

What does the patient do when the pain occurs? How does it affect activity? School attendance, school stress, school phobia. What fears does the child have? What activities has the child discontinued?

Past Testing: Endoscopies, x-rays, upper GI series.

Past Medical History: Diabetes, asthma, surgery, diabetes, prematurity. Prior treatment for a abdominal pain.

Family History: Abdominal pain in family members, urolithiasis, migraine, peptic ulcer disease, irritable bowel syndrome, hemolytic anemia, chronic pain.

Social History: Recent travel, change in schools, change in water and food consumption, marital discord, recent losses (grandparent, pet), general family function. Review of a typical day, including meals, activities, sleep pattern, school schedule, time of bowel movements; drugs/alcohol, sexual activity, sexual abuse.

Review of Systems: Growth, weight gain, stool pattern, bloating, distension, hematemesis, hematochezia, jaundice. Headache, limb pain, dizziness, fatigue, weakness. Stress- or tension-related symptoms.

Physical Examination

General Appearance: Degree of distress, septic appearance. Note whether the patient looks "ill" or well.

Vitals: Temperature (fever), pulse (tachycardia), BP (hypertension, hypotension), respiratory rate (tachypnea). Growth percentiles, deceleration in growth, weight-for-height.

Skin: Pallor, rashes, nodules, jaundice, purpura, petechia.

HEENT: Pale conjunctiva, scleral icterus.

Lymph Nodes: Cervical, periumbilical, inguinal lymphadenopathy, Virchow node (enlarged supraclavicular node).

Chest: Breath sounds, rhonchi, wheeze.

Heart: Murmurs, distant heart sounds, peripheral pulses.

Abdomen

  Inspection: Abdominal distention, scars, visible peristalsis.

  Auscultation: Quality and pattern of bowel sounds; high-pitched bowel sounds (partial obstruction), bruits.

  Palpation: Palpation while noting the patient's appearance, reaction, and distractibility. Tenderness, rebound, masses, hepatomegaly; liver texture (smooth, coarse), splenomegaly; retained fecal material. Bimanual palpation of flank (nephromegaly), hernias (inguinal, femoral, umbilical); costovertebral angle tenderness.

    McBurney's point tenderness: Located two thirds of the way between umbilicus and anterior superior iliac spine, appendicitis.

    Rovsing's sign: Manual pressure and release at left lower quadrant causes referred pain at McBurney's point, appendicitis.

  Percussion: Tympany, liver and spleen span by percussion.

Perianal Examination: Fissures, fistulas, hemorrhoids, skin tags, underwear soiling (fecal or urinary incontinence).

Rectal Examination: Impacted stool, masses, tenderness; gross or occult blood.

Male Genital Examination: Hernias, undescended testes, hypospadias.

Female Genital Examination: Hymeneal ring trauma, imperforate hymen, urethra, distal vagina. Pelvic examination in pubertal girls. Cervical discharge, adnexal tenderness, masses, cervical motion tenderness.

Extremities: Brachial pulses, femoral pulses, edema. Digital clubbing, loss of nailbed angle (osteoarthropathy).

Neurologic Examination: Observation of the patient moving on and off of the examination table; gait.

Laboratory Evaluation: CBC, electrolytes, BUN, liver function tests, amylase, lipase, UA, pregnancy test.

Chest X-ray: Free air under diaphragm, infiltrates.

X-rays of Abdomen (acute abdomen series): Flank stripe, subdiaphragmatic free air, distended loops of bowel, air fluid levels, mass effects, calcifications, fecaliths.

Differential Diagnosis of Recurrent Abdominal Pain

Gastrointestinal Causes
Antral gastritis, peptic ulcer
Constipation
Crohn disease
Carbohydrate malabsorption
Pancreatitis
Cholelithiasis
Malrotation and volvulus
Intestinal parasitic infection (G. lamblia)
Urinary Tract Disorders
Ureteropelvic junction obstruction
Urinary tract infection
Urolithiasis

Psychogenic Causes
Conversion reaction
Somatization disorder
Anxiety disorder
Other Causes
Intervertebral disk disease
Spine disease
Musculoskeletal trauma
Migraine or cyclic vomiting
Abdominal epilepsy

Persistent Vomiting

Chief Complaint: Vomiting.

History of Present Illness: Character of emesis (effortless, forceful, projectile, color, food, uncurdled milk, bilious, feculent, blood, coffee ground material); abdominal pain, retching, fever, headache, cough.

Jaundice, recent change in medications. Ingestion of spoiled food; exposure to ill contacts. Overfeeding, weight and growth parameters, vigorous hand or finger sucking, maternal polyhydramnios. Wheezing, irritability, apnea.

Emesis related to meals; specific foods that induce emesis (food allergy or intolerance to milk, soy, gluten). Pain on swallowing (odynophagia), difficulty swallowing (dysphagia). Diarrhea, constipation.

Proper formula preparation, air gulping, postcibal handling. Constant headache, worse with Valsalva maneuver and occurring with morning emesis (increased ICP).

Possibility of pregnancy (last menstrual period, contraception, sexual history). Prior X-rays, upper GI series, endoscopy.

Past Medical History: Diabetes, peptic ulcer, CNS disease. Travel, animal or pet exposure.

Medications: Digoxin, theophylline, chemotherapy, anticholinergics, morphine, ergotamines, oral contraceptives, progesterone, erythromycin.

Family History: Migraine headaches.

Historical Findings in Persistent Vomiting

Appearance of Vomitus
  Large volume, bilious
  Uncurdled milk, food
  Bile
  Feculent emesis
  Bloody, coffee-grounds
Character of Emetic Act
  Effortless, nonbilious
  Tongue thrusting
  Finger sucking, gagging
  Projectile vomiting
Timing of Emesis
  Early morning
  Related to meals or foods

Other Gastrointestinal Symptoms
  Nausea
  Swallowing difficulties
  Constipation
  Pain
  Jaundice
Neurologic Symptoms
  Headache
  Seizures
General
  Respiratory distress
  Travel, animal/pet exposure
  Ill family members
  Stress

Physical Examination

General Appearance: Signs of dehydration, septic appearance. Note whether the patient looks "ill" or well.

Vital Signs: BP (hypotension, hypertension), pulse (tachycardia), respiratory rate, temperature (fever). Growth percentiles.

Skin: Pallor, jaundice, flushing, rash.

HEENT: Nystagmus, papilledema; ketone odor on breath (apple odor, diabetic ketoacidosis); jugular venous distention. Bulging fontanelle, papilledema.

Lungs: Wheezes, rhonchi, rales.

Abdomen: Tenderness to percussion, distention, increased bowel sounds, rebound tenderness (peritonitis). Nephromegaly, masses, hepatomegaly, splenomegaly, costovertebral angle tenderness.

Extremities: Edema, cyanosis.

Genitourinary: Adnexal tenderness, uterine enlargement.

Rectal: Perirectal lesions, localized tenderness, masses, occult blood.

Neurologic Examination: Strength, sensation, posture, gait, deep tendon reflexes.

Physical Examination Findings in Persistent Vomiting

Vital Signs: Tachycardia, bradycardia, tachypnea, fever, hypotension, hypertension, short stature, poor weight gain
Abdomen
  Distention
  Absent bowel sounds
  Increased bowel sounds
  Rebound tenderness
  Masses

Genitourinary System
  Adnexal pain
  Mass
  Rectal mass
Respiratory: Bronchospasm, pneumonia
Neurologic: Migraine, seizures, increased intracranial pressure
Renal: Flank pain
Skin: Rash, purpura

Laboratory Evaluation: CBC, electrolytes, UA, amylase, lipase, LFTs, pregnancy test, abdominal X-ray series.

Differential Diagnosis of Vomiting in Infants Under 2 Weeks of Age

Functional
 Innocent vomiting
 Gastroesophageal reflux
 Postcibal handling
 Improper formula preparation
 Aerophagia
Gastrointestinal Obstruction
 Esophageal: obstruction atresia, stenosis, vascular ring, tracheal
 esophageal fistula, cricopharyngeal incoordination, achalasia, natal hernia,
 diaphragmatic hernia
Torsion of the stomach
Malrotation of the bowel
Volvulus
Intestinal atresia, stenosis, meconium ileus with cystic fibrosis, meconium plug
Webs
Annular pancreas
Paralytic ileus (peritonitis, postoperative, acute infection, hypokalemia)
 Hirschsprung disease
 Imperforate anus
 Enteric duplication

Other gastrointestinal causes: Necrotizing enterocolitis, congenital lactose
 intolerance, milk-soy protein intolerance, lactobeazor, GI perforation,
 hepatitis, pancreatitis
Neurologic: Increased intracranial pressure, subdural hydrocephalus, edema,
 kernicterus
Renal: Obstructive uropathy, renal insufficiency
Infection: Systemic infections, pyelonephritis
Metabolic: Urea cycle deficiencies, aminoacidopathies, disorders of carbohydrate
 metabolism, acidosis, congenital adrenal hyperplasia, tetany, hypercalcemia
Drugs/toxins: Theophylline, caffeine, digoxin
Blood: Swallowed maternal blood, gastritis, ulcers
Pneumonia
Dysautonomia
Postoperative anesthesia

Differential Diagnosis of Vomiting in Infants 2 Weeks to 12 Months of Age

Gastroesophageal reflux, esophagitis

Functional
  Innocent
  Improper formula preparation
  Aerophagia
  Postcibal handling
  Nervous
  Rumination

Esophageal: Foreign body, stenosis, vascular ring, tracheoesophageal fistula cricopharyngeal incoordination, achalasia, hiatal hernia

Stomach: Bezoar, lactobeazor

Intestinal obstruction, pyloric stenosis, malrotation, Meckel diverticulitis, intussusception, incarcerated hernia, Hirschsprung disease, appendicitis, intestinal duplications

Other gastrointestinal causes: Annular pancreas, paralytic ileus, hypokalemia, Helicobacter sp. infection, peritonitis, pancreatitis, celiac disease, viral and bacterial enteritis, lactose intolerance, milk-soy protein intolerance, cholecystitis, gallstones, pseudo-obstruction

Neurologic: Increased intracranial (subdural hematoma, hydrocephalus, cerebral edema)

Renal: Obstructive uropathy, renal insufficiency, stones

Infectious: Meningitis, sepsis, pyelonephritis, otitis media, sinusitis, pertussis, hepatitis, parasitic infestation

Metabolic: Urea cycle deficiencies, aminoacidopathies, disorder of carbohydrate metabolism, acidosis, congenital adrenal hyperplasia, tetany, hypercalcemia

Drugs/toxins: Theophylline, digoxin, iron, ipecac

Blood

Hydrometrocolpos

Radiation/chemotherapy

Reye syndrome

Psychogenic vomiting

Munchausen syndrome by proxy

Differential Diagnosis of Vomiting in Children Older Than 12 Months of Age

Gastroesophageal reflux
Gastrointestinal obstruction
  Esophagea: Esophagitis, foreign body, corrosive ingestion, hiatal hernia
  Stomach: Foreign body, bezoar, chronic granulomatous disease
  Intestinal obstruction: Pyloric channel ulcer, intramural hematoma, malrotation, volvulus, Meckel diverticulitis, meconium ileus in cystic fibrosis, incarcerated hernia, intussusception, Hirschsprung disease, ulcerative colitis, Crohn disease, superior mesenteric artery syndrome
Other gastrointestinal causes: Annular pancreas, paralytic ileus, hypokalemia, Helicobacter pylori infection, peritonitis, pancreatitis, celiac disease, viral or bacterial enteritis, hepatobiliary disease, gallstone ileus, Henoch-Schönlein purpura.
Neurologic: Increased intracranial pressure, Leigh disease, migraine, motion sickness, seizures
Renal: Obstructive uropathy, renal insufficiency, stones
Infection: Meningitis, sepsis, pyelonephritis, otitis media, sinusitis, hepatitis, parasitic infestation, streptococcal pharyngitis, labyrinthitis
Metabolic: Inborn errors of metabolism, acidosis, diabetic ketoacidosis, adrenal insufficiency
Drugs/toxins: Aspirin, digoxin, iron, lead, ipecac, elicit drugs
Torsion of the testis or ovary
Blood
Radiation/chemotherapy
Reye syndrome
Postoperative vomiting
Cyclic vomiting
Pregnancy
Psychologic: Bulimia nervosa, anorexia nervosa, stress, Munchausen syndrome by proxy

Jaundice and Hepatitis

Chief Complaint: Jaundice.
History of Present Illness: Timing, progression, distribution of jaundice. Abdominal pain, anorexia, vomiting, fever, dark urine, pruritus, arthralgias, rash, diarrhea. Gradual, caudal progression of jaundice (physiologic jaundice or breast-feeding jaundice), blood products, raw shellfish, day care centers, foreign travel.
Past Medical History: Hepatitis serologies, liver function tests, liver biopsy, hepatitis immunization.
Perinatal History: Course of the pregnancy, illnesses, infections, medications taken during the pregnancy. Inability to pass meconium (cystic fibrosis), failure to thrive, irritability. Newborn hypoglycemia, lethargy after the first formula feedings (carbohydrate metabolic disorders).
Medications: Acetaminophen, isoniazid, phenytoin.
Family History: Liver disease, familial jaundice, lung disease, alpha$_1$-antitrypsin deficiency. History of perinatal infant death (metabolic disorders).
Social History: IV drug abuse, alcohol, exposure to hepatitis.

Historical Findings in Jaundice	
Neonate	**Older Child**
Family history: Familial jaundice, emphysema, infant deaths **Prenatal history:** Infection in pregnancy, maternal risk for hepatitis, medications **Perinatal history:** Hypoglycemia, vomiting, lethargy with feedings, failure to pass meconium, icterus, acholic stools.	**Acute illness** **Failure to thrive** **Family history of jaundice** **Exposure:** Blood products, raw shellfish, travel, drug abuse

Physical Examination

General Appearance: Signs of dehydration, septic appearance, irritability. Note whether the patient looks "ill" or well.

Vital Signs: Pulse, BP, respiratory rate, temperature (fever).

Skin: Ecchymoses, excoriations, jaundice, urticaria, bronze discoloration (hemochromatosis), diffuse rash (perinatal infection). Malar rash, discord lesions (lupus), erythematous scaling papules (cystic fibrosis).

Lymph Nodes: Cervical or inguinal lymphadenopathy.

Head: Cephalohematoma, hypertelorism, high forehead, large fontanelle, pursed lips (Zellweger syndrome), microcephaly.

Eyes: Scleral icterus, cataracts, Kayser-Fleischer rings (bronze corneal pigmentation, Wilson's disease), xanthomas (chronic liver disease).

Mouth: Sublingual jaundice.

Heart: Rhythm, murmurs.

Chest: Gynecomastia, breath sounds.

Abdomen: Bowel sounds, bruits, right upper quadrant tenderness; liver span, hepatomegaly; liver margin texture (blunt, irregular, firm, smooth), splenomegaly; ascites.

Extremities: Joint tenderness, joint swelling, palmar erythema, edema, anasarca. Jaundice, erythematous nodules over shins (erythema nodosum).

Neurologic: Lethargy, hypotonia, neuromuscular deficits.

Rectal: Perianal skin tags (inflammatory bowel disease), hemorrhoids, occult blood.

Laboratory Evaluation of Jaundice

Screening Labs
Complete blood count, platelets, differential, smear
AST, ALT, GGT, alkaline phosphatase
Total and fractionated bilirubin
Protein, albumin levels
INR, PTT
Stool color

Assessment Labs
Infection
  Cultures of blood, urine, cerebrospinal fluid
  Serologies: Toxoplasmosis, rubella, cytomegalovirus, herpes, hepatitis panel, syphilis, Epstein-Barr virus
Metabolic
  Alpha$_1$-antitrypsin level and Pi typing
  Thyroxine and thyroid stimulating hormone
  Metabolic screen: Urine/serum amino acids
  Sweat chloride test
  Ceruloplasmin, urinary copper excretion
  Toxicology screen
Structural
  24-hour duodenal intubation for bilirubin excretion
  Ultrasound
  Radionuclide or hepatobiliary scan
  Operative cholangiogram
Autoimmune/inflammatory: ESR, ANA

Pathologic Diagnosis
Liver biopsy
Bone marrow biopsy (enzyme deficiency, hemoglobinopathies, hemolytic anemias)

Differential Diagnosis of Neonatal Jaundice

Nonpathologic Causes
Physiologic jaundice
Breast milk jaundice
Pathologic Causes
Unconjugated hyperbilirubinemia
Bilirubin overproduction
    ABO/Rh incompatibility
    Hemoglobinopathies
    Erythrocyte membrane defects
    Polycythemia
    Extravascular blood
Increased uptake
    Increased enterohepatic uptake
    Intestinal obstruction
Genetic
    Crigler-Najjar types I and II
    Gilbert syndrome
Miscellaneous
    Hypothyroidism
    Sepsis, urinary tract infection
    Hypoxia, acidosis
    Hypoglycemia
    Maternal diabetes mellitus
    High intestinal obstruction
    Drugs
    Fatty acids (hyperalimentation)
    Lucy-Driscoll syndrome
Conjugated hyperbilirubinemia
Anatomic
    Extrahepatic
        Biliary atresia
        Bile duct stenosis
        Choledochal cyst
        Bile duct perforation
        Biliary sludge
        Biliary stone or neoplasm
    Intrahepatic
        Alagille syndrome
        Nonsyndromic interlobular ductal
        hypoplasia
        Caroli disease
        Congenital hepatic fibrosis
        Inspissated bile

Conjugated hyperbilirubinemia (continued)
Metabolic/genetic
    Alpha,-antitrypsin deficiency
    Galactosemia
    Fructose intolerance
    Glycogen storage disease
    Tyrosinemia
    Zellweger syndrome
    Cystic fibrosis
Excretory defects
    Dubin-Johnson syndrome
    Rotor syndrome
    Summerskill syndrome
    Byler disease
Infections
    TORCH (toxoplasmosis, other
        agents, rubella, cytomegalovirus,
        herpes simplex)
    Syphilis
    HIV
    Varicella-zoster virus
    Coxsackievirus
    Hepatitis (A, B, C, D, and E)
    Echovirus
    Tuberculosis
    Gram-negative infections
    Listeria monocytogenes
    Staphylococcus aureus
    Sepsis, urinary tract infections
Miscellaneous
    Trisomies 17, 18, 21
    Total parenteral nutrition
    Postoperative jaundice
    Extracorporeal membrane oxygenation
    Idiopathic neonatal hepatitis

Differential Diagnosis of Jaundice in Older Children	

Metabolic/Genetic
Gilbert syndrome
Dubin-Johnson syndrome
Rotor syndrome
Cystic fibrosis
Indian childhood cirrhosis
Wilson disease
Tyrosinemia
Alpha$_1$-antitrypsin deficiency
 	
Anatomic
Caroli disease
Congenital hepatic fibrosis
Choledochal cyst
Cholelithiasis
Pancreas and pancreatic duct
abnormalities
Infections
Viral
  Hepatitis (A, B, C, D, E), CMV
  Epstein-Barr virus
	Infections (continued)
	Viral
	  Herpes simplex virus
	  Varicella-zoster virus
	  Adenovirus
	  Enterovirus
	  Rubella virus
	  Arbovirus
	  HIV
	  Echovirus
	Bacterial
	  Sepsis
	  Toxic shock syndrome
	  Lyme disease
	  Rocky mountain spotted
	  fever
	Miscellaneous
	  Visceral larval migrans
	  Schistosomiasis
	  Reye syndrome

Hepatosplenomegaly

Chief Complaint: Liver or spleen enlarged.

History of Present Illness: Duration of enlargement of the liver or spleen. Acute or chronic illness, fever, jaundice, pallor, bruising, weight loss, fatigue, joint pain, joint stiffness. Nutritional history, growth delay. Neurodevelopmental delay or loss of developmental milestones.

Past Medical History: Previous organomegaly, neurologic symptoms. General health.

Perinatal History: Prenatal complications, neonatal jaundice.

Medications: Current and past drugs, anticonvulsants, toxins.

Family History: Storage diseases, metabolic disorders, hepatic fibrosis, alpha$_1$-antitrypsin deficiency. History of neonatal death.

Social History: Infections, toxin, exposures, drugs or alcohol.

Physical Examination

General Appearance: Wasting, ill appearance, malnutrition.

Vital Signs: Blood pressure, temperature, pulse, respirations. Growth curve.

HEENT: Head size and shape, icterus, cataracts (galactosemia), Kayser-Fleischer rings (Wilson disease). Coarsening of facial features (mucopolysaccharidoses).

Skin: Excoriations, spider angiomas (chronic liver disease, bilary obstruction of the biliary tract); pallor, petechiae, bruising (malignancy, chronic liver disease); erythema nodosum (inflammatory bowel disease, sarcoidosis).

Lymph Nodes: Location and size of lymphadenopathy.

Lungs: Crackles, wheeze, rhonchi.

Abdomen: Distension, prominent superficial veins (portal hypertension), umbilical hernia, bruits. Percussion of flanks for shifting dullness. Liver span by percussion, hepatomegaly. Liver consistency and texture. Spleen size and texture, splenomegaly.

Perianal: Hemorrhoids (portal hypertension), fissures, skin tags, fistulas (inflammatory bowel disease).

Rectal Exam: Masses, tenderness.

Extremities: Edema, joint tenderness, joint swelling, joint erythema (juvenile rheumatoid arthritis, mucopolysaccharidoses). Clubbing (hypoxia, intestinal disorders, hepatic disorders).

Physical Examination Findings in Hepatosplenomegaly

Growth curve failure
Skin: Icterus, pallor, edema, pruritus, spider nevi, petechiae and bruises, rashes
Head--microcephaly or macrocephaly
Eyes--cataracts (galactosemia); Kayser-Fleischer rings (Wilson disease)
Nodes--generalized lymphadenopathy
Chest--adventitious sounds
Heart--gallop, tachycardia, rub, pulsus paradoxus
Abdomen--ascites, large kidneys, prominent veins, hepatosplenomegaly
Rectal--hemorrhoids, sphincter tone, fissures, fistulas, skin tags with inflammatory
   bowel disease
Neurologic-- developmental delay, dystonia, tremor, absent reflexes, ataxia

---

Differential Diagnosis of Hepatosplenomegaly

Predominant Splenomegaly	Predominant Hepatomegaly
Infection Viral–Epstein-Barr, cytomegalovirus, parvovirus B19 Bacterial--endocarditis, shunt infection Protozoal--malaria, babesiosis *Hematologic* Hemolytic anemias Porphyrias Osteopetrosis, myelofibrosis *Vascular* Portal vein anomalies Hepatic scarring or fibrosis *Tumor and infiltration* Cysts, hemangiomas, hamartomas Lymphoreticular malignancies Neuroblastoma	CMV, syphilis, neonatal hepatitis Hepatitis--A, B, C, D, E, tuberculosis, sarcoidosis, chronic granulomatous disease Drugs--alcohol, phenytoin Sclerosing cholangitis, infectious cholangitis Abscess Chronic active hepatitis Cardiac--failure, pericarditis Budd-Chiari syndrome Paroxysmal nocturnal hemoglobinuria Biliary atresia or hypoplasia Choledochal cyst Congenital hepatic fibrosis Child abuse--trauma Galactosemia, glycogen storage disease, fructose intolerance Tyrosinemia, urea cycle disorders Cystic fibrosis Alpha$_1$-antitrypsin deficiency Wilson disease, hemochromatosis Fatty change: Malnutrition, obesity, alcohol, corticosteroids, diabetes Primary or metastatic tumors

Acute Diarrhea

Chief Complaint: Diarrhea.

History of Present Illness: Duration and frequency, of diarrhea; number of stools per day, characteristics of stools (bloody, mucus, watery, formed, oily, foul odor); fever, abdominal pain or cramps, flatulence, anorexia, vomiting. Season (rotavirus occurs in the winter). Amount of fluid intake and food intake.

Past Medical History: Recent ingestion of spoiled poultry (salmonella), spoiled milk, seafood (shrimp, shellfish; Vibrio parahaemolyticus); common food sources (restaurants), travel history. Ill contacts with diarrhea, sexual exposures.

Family History: Coeliac disease.

Medications Associated with Diarrhea: Magnesium-containing antacids, laxatives, antibiotics.

Immunizations: Rotavirus immunization.

Physical Examination

General Appearance: Signs of dehydration. Note whether the patient looks septic, well, or malnourished.

Vital Signs: BP(hypotension), pulse (tachycardia), respiratory rate, temperature (fever).

Skin: Turgor, delayed capillary refill, jaundice.

HEENT: Dry mucous membranes.

Chest: Breath sounds.

Heart: Rhythm, gallops, murmurs.

Abdomen: Distention, high-pitched rushes, tenderness, splenomegaly, hepatomegaly.

Extremities: Joint swelling, edema.

Rectal: Sphincter tone, guaiac test.

Laboratory Evaluation: Electrolytes, CBC with differential. Gram's stain of stool for leukocytes. Cultures for enteric pathogens, stool for ova and parasites x 3; stool and blood for clostridium difficile toxin; blood cultures.

Stool occult blood. Stool cultures for cholera, E. coli 0157:H7, Yersinia; rotavirus assay.

Differential Diagnosis of Acute Diarrhea: Rotavirus, Norwalk virus, salmonella, shigella, E coli, Campylobacter, Bacillus cereus, traveler's diarrhea, antibiotic-related diarrhea.

Chronic Diarrhea

Chief Complaint: Diarrhea.

History of Present Illness: Duration, frequency, and timing of diarrheal episodes. Volume of stool output (number of stools per day). Effect of fasting on diarrhea. Prior dietary manipulations and their effect on stooling. Formula changes, fever, abdominal pain, flatulence, tenesmus (painful urge to defecate), anorexia, vomiting, myalgias, arthralgias, weight loss, rashes.

Stool Appearance: Watery, formed, blood or mucus, oily, foul odor.

Travel history, laxative abuse, inflammatory bowel disease. Sexual exposures, AIDS risk factors. Exacerbation by stress.

Past Medical History: Pattern of stooling from birth. Growth deficiency, weight gain. Three-day dietary record, ill contacts.

Medications and Substances Associated with Diarrhea: Laxatives, magnesium-containing antacids, cholinergic agents, milk (lactase deficiency), gum (sorbitol).

Family History: Family members with diarrhea, milk intolerance, coeliac disease.

Social History: Water supply, meal preparation, sanitation, pet or animal exposures.

Historical Findings in Chronic Diarrhea	
Age of onset Stool characteristics Diet (new food/formula) Growth delay Family history of allergy; genetic, metabolic, or inborn errors	Secretory symptoms: Large volume, watery diarrhea Osmotic symptoms: Large numbers of soft stools Systemic symptoms: Fever, nausea, malaise

Physical Examination

General Appearance: Signs of dehydration or malnutrition. Septic appearance. Note whether the patient looks "ill," well, or malnourished.

Vital Signs: Growth percentiles, pulse (tachycardia), respiratory rate, temperature (fever), blood pressure (hypertension, neuroblastoma; hypotension, dehydration).

Skin: Turgor, delayed capillary refill, jaundice, pallor (anemia), hair thinning, rashes, erythema nodosum, pyoderma gangrenosum, maculopapular rashes (inflammatory bowel disease), hyperpigmentation (adrenal insufficiency).

Eyes: Bitot spots (vitamin A deficiency), adenopathy.

Mouth: Oral ulcers (Crohn disease, coeliac disease), dry mucous membranes; cheilosis (cracked lips, riboflavin deficiency); glossitis (B12, folate deficiency); oropharyngeal candidiasis (AIDS).

Lymph Nodes: Cervical, axillary, inguinal lymphadenopathy.

Chest: Thoracic shape, crackles, wheezing.

Abdomen: Distention (malnutrition), hyperactive, bowel sounds, tenderness, masses, palpable bowel loops, palpable stool. Hepatomegaly, splenomegaly.

Extremities: Joint tenderness, swelling (ulcerative colitis); gluteal wasting (malnutrition), dependent edema.

Genitalia: Signs of child abuse or sexual activity.

Perianal Examination: Skin tags and fistulas.

Rectal: Perianal or rectal ulcers, sphincter tone, tenderness, masses, impacted stool, occult blood, sphincter reflex.

Neurologic: Mental status changes, peripheral neuropathy (B6, B12 deficiency), decreased perianal sensation. Ataxia, diminished deep tendon reflexes, decreased proprioception.

Physical Examination Findings in Chronic Diarrhea

Poor growth	Clubbing
Hypertension	Lung crackles, wheezing
Fever	Abdominal mass
Jaundice	Organomegaly
Rash	Abnormal genitalia
Erythema nodosum	Perianal tags
Pyoderma gangrenosa	Rectal impaction
Edema	Ataxia, decreased deep tendon reflexes

Laboratory Evaluation: Electrolytes, CBC with differential. Wright's stain for fecal leucocytes; cultures for enteric pathogens, ova and parasites x 3; clostridium difficile toxin. Stool carbohydrate content. Stool for occult blood, neutral fat (maldigestion); split fat (malabsorption).

Differential Diagnosis of Chronic Diarrhea

Small Infants and Babies
Chronic nonspecific diarrhea of infancy/postinfectious diarrhea
Milk and soy protein intolerance
Protracted infectious enteritis
Microvillous inclusion disease
Celiac disease
Hirschsprung's disease
Congenital transport defects
Nutrient malabsorption
Munchausen's syndrome by proxy

Toddlers
Chronic nonspecific diarrhea
Protracted viral enteritis
Giardiasis
Sucrase isomaltase deficiency
Tumors (secretotory diarrhea)
Celiac disease
Ulcerative colitis

School-Aged Children
Inflammatory bowel disease
Appendiceal abscess
Lactase deficiency
Constipation with encopresis
Laxative abuse
Giardiasis

Constipation

Chief Complaint: Constipation.

History of Present Illness: Stool frequency, consistency, size; stooling pattern birth to the present. Encopresis, bulky, fatty stools, foul odor. Hard stools, painful defecation, straining, streaks of blood on stools. Dehydration, urinary incontinence, enuresis. Abdominal pain, fever. Recent change in diet. Soiling characteristics and time of day. Are stools formed or scybalous (small, dry, rabbit-like pellets)? Withholding behavior.

Dietary History: Excessive cow's milk or limited fiber consumption; breast-feeding.

Past Medical History: Recent illness, bed rest, fever.

Medications Associated with Constipation: Opiate analgesics, aluminum-containing antacids, iron supplements, antihistamines, antidepressants.

Social History: Recent birth of a sibling, emotional stress, housing move.

Family History: Constipation.

Physical Examination

General Appearance: Dehydration or malnutrition. Septic appearance, weak cry. Note whether the patient looks "ill," well, or malnourished.

Vital Signs: BP (hypertension, pheochromocytoma), pulse, respiratory rate, temperature. Growth percentiles, poor growth.

Skin: Café au lait spots (neurofibromatosis), jaundice.

Eyes: Decreased pupillary response, icterus.

Mouth: Cheilosis (cracked lips, riboflavin deficiency), oral ulcers (inflammatory bowel, coeliac disease), dry mucous membranes, glossitis (B12, folate deficiency), oropharyngeal candidiasis (AIDS).

Abdomen: Distention, peristaltic waves, weak abdominal musculature (muscular dystrophy, prune-belly syndrome). Hyperactive bowel sounds, tenderness, hepatomegaly. Palpable stool, fecal masses above the pubic symphysis and in the left lower quadrant.

Perianal: Anterior ectopic anus, anterior anal displacement. Anal fissures, excoriation, dermatitis, perianal ulcers. Rectal prolapse. Soiling in the perianal area. Sphincter reflex: Gentle rubbing of the perianal skin results in reflex contraction of the external anal sphincter.

Rectal: Sphincter tone, rectal ulcers, tenderness, hemorrhoids, masses. Stool in a cavernous ampulla, occult blood.

Extremities: Joint tenderness, joint swelling (ulcerative colitis).

Neurologic: Developmental delay, mental retardation, peripheral neuropathy (B6, B12 deficiency), decreased perianal sensation.

Laboratory Evaluation: Electrolytes, CBC with differential, calcium.

Abdominal X-ray: Air fluid levels, dilation, pancreatic calcifications.

Differential Diagnosis of Constipation in Neonates and Young Infants

Meconium ileus
Meconium plug syndrome
Functional ileus of the newborn
Small left colon syndrome
Volvulus
Intestinal web
Intestinal stenosis
Intestinal atresia
Intestinal stricture (necrotizing
    enterocolitis)
Imperforate anus
Anal stenosis
Anterior ectopic anus
Anterior anal displacement

Hirschsprung disease
Acquired aganglionosis
Tumors
Myelodysplasia
Hypothyroidism
Maternal opiates
Inadequate nutrition/fluids
Excessive cow's milk consumption
Absence of abdominal musculature
    (prune-belly syndrome)
Cerebral palsy

Differential Diagnosis of Constipation in Older Infants and Children

Physiologic Causes
Breast milk, cow's milk, low roughage
Deficient fluid: Fever, heat, immobility,
    anorexia nervosa
Voluntary Stool Withholding
Megacolon
Painful defecation: Anal fissure,
    perianal dermatitis, hemorrhoids
Behavioral issues
Mental retardation
Neurogenic Disorders
Hirschsprung disease
Intestinal pseudoobstruction
Cerebral palsy
Myelomeningocele
Spinal cord injury
Transverse myelitis
Spinal dysraphism
Neurofibromatosis
Myopathies
Rickets
Prune-belly syndrome

Endocrine and Metabolic Disorders
Hypothyroidism
Diabetes mellitus
Pheochromocytoma
Hypokalemia
Hypercalcemia
Hypocalcemia
Diabetes insipidus
Renal tubular acidosis
Porphyria
Amyloidosis
Lipid storage disorders
Miscellaneous Disorders
Anal or rectal stenosis
Anteriorly placed anus
Appendicitis
Celiac disease
Scleroderma
Lead poisoning
Viral hepatitis
Salmonellosis
Tetanus
Chagas disease
Drugs

Hematemesis and Upper Gastrointestinal Bleeding

Chief Complaint: Vomiting blood.

History of Present Illness: Duration and frequency of hematemesis, characteristics of vomitus (bright red blood, coffee ground material), volume of blood, hematocrit. Forceful retching prior to hematemesis (Mallory-Weiss tear).

Abdominal pain, melena, hematochezia; peptic ulcer, prior bleeding episodes, nose bleeds. Weight loss, anorexia, jaundice; bright red foods, drinks.

Past Medical History: Diabetes, bleeding disorders, renal failure, liver disease. Gastrointestinal surgery.

Medications: Alcohol, aspirin, nonsteroidal anti-inflammatory drugs, anticoagulants, steroids.

Physical Examination

General Appearance: Pallor, diaphoresis, confusion, dehydration. Note whether the patient looks "ill," well, or malnourished.

Vital Signs: Supine and upright pulse and blood pressure (orthostatic hypotension) (resting tachycardia indicates a 10-20% blood volume loss; postural hypotension indicates a 20-30% blood loss), temperature.

Skin: Delayed capillary refill, pallor, petechiae. Hemorrhagic telangiectasia (Osler-Weber-Rendu syndrome), abnormal pigmentation (Peutz-Jeghers syndrome), jaundice, ecchymoses (coagulopathy), increased skin elasticity (Ehlers-Danlos syndrome).

Eyes: Scleral pallor.

Mouth: Oropharyngeal lacerations, nasal bleeding, labial and buccal pigmentation (Peutz-Jeghers syndrome).

Chest: Gynecomastia, breath sounds.

Heart: Systolic ejection murmur.

Abdomen: Dilated abdominal veins, bowel sounds, distention, tenderness, masses, hepatic atrophy, splenomegaly.

Extremities: Edema, cold extremities.

Neurologic: Decreased mental status, gait.

Rectal: Masses, hemorrhoids. Polyps, fissures; stool color, occult blood testing.

Laboratory Evaluation: CBC, platelet count, reticulocyte count, international normalized ratio (INR), partial thromboplastin time (PTT), bleeding time, electrolytes, BUN, creatinine, glucose. Type and cross-match for 2-4 units of packed RBC and transfuse as needed. ALT, AST, GGTP, glucose, electrolytes. Esophagogastroduodenoscopy, colonoscopy, Meckel's scan, bleeding scan.

Differential Diagnosis of Upper Gastrointestinal Bleeding		
Age	**Common**	**Less Common**
Neonates (0-30 days)	Swallowed maternal blood, gastritis, duodenitis	Coagulopathy, vascular malformations, gastric/esophageal duplication, leiomyoma
Infants (30 days-1 year)	Gastritis, gastric ulcer, esophagitis, duodenitis	Esophageal varices, foreign body, aortoesophageal fistula
Children (1-12 years)	Esophagitis, esophageal varices, gastritis, gastric ulcer, duodenal ulcer, Mallory-Weiss tear, nasopharyngeal bleeding	Leiomyoma, salicylates, vascular malformation, hematobilia, NSAIDs

Age	Common	Less Common
Adolescents (12 years-adult)	Duodenal ulcer, esopha-gitis, esophageal varices, gastritis, Mallory-Weiss tear	Thrombocytopenia, Dieula-foy's ulcer, hematobilia

Melena and Lower Gastrointestinal Bleeding

Chief Complaint: Anal bleeding
History of Present Illness: Duration, quantity, color of bleeding (gross blood, streaks on stool, melena), recent hematocrit. Change in bowel habits, change in stool caliber, abdominal pain, fever. Constipation, diarrhea, anorectal pain. Epistaxis, anorexia, weight loss, malaise, vomiting.
Fecal mucus, excessive straining during defecation. Colitis, peptic ulcer, hematemesis.
Past Medical History: Barium enema, colonoscopy, sigmoidoscopy, upper GI series.
Medications: Anticoagulants, aspirin, NSAIDs.

Physical Examination
General Appearance: Dehydration, pallor. Note whether the patient looks ill, well, or malnourished.
Vital Signs: BP (orthostatic hypotension), pulse, respiratory rate, temperature (tachycardia).
Skin: Delayed capillary refill, pallor, jaundice. Spider angiomata, rashes, purpura.
Eyes: Pale conjunctiva, icterus.
Mouth: Buccal mucosa discolorations or pigmentation (Henoch-Schönlein purpura or Peutz-Jeghers syndrome).
Chest: Breath sounds.
Heart: Systolic ejection murmurs.
Abdomen: Masses, distention, tenderness, hernias, liver atrophy, splenomegaly.
Genitourinary: Testicular atrophy.
Extremities: Cold, pale extremities.
Neurologic: Anxiety, confusion.
Rectal: Hemorrhoids, masses; fissures, polyps, ulcers. Gross or occult blood.
Laboratory Evaluation: CBC (anemia), liver function tests. Abdominal x-ray series (thumbprinting, air fluid levels).

Differential Diagnosis of Lower Gastrointestinal Bleeding		
Age	Common	Less Common
Neonates (0-30 days)	Anorectal lesions, swal-lowed maternal blood, milk allergy, necrotizing enterocolitis, midgut volvulus	Vascular malformations, Hirschsprung's entero-colitis, intestinal duplica-tion, coagulopathy

Age	Common	Less Common
Infants (30 days- 1 year)	Anorectal lesions, midgut volvulus, intussusception (under 3 years) Meckel's diverticulitis, infectious diarrhea, milk protein allergy	Vascular malformations, intestinal duplication, acquired thrombocytopenia
Children (1-12 years)	Juvenile polyps, Meckel's diverticulitis, intussusception (under 3 years), infectious diarrhea, anal fissure, nodular lymphoid hyperplasia	Henoch-Schönlein purpura, hemolytic-uremic syndrome, vasculitis (SLE), inflammatory bowel disease
Adolescents (12 years-adult)	Inflammatory bowel disease, polyps, hemorrhoids, anal fissure, infectious diarrhea	Arteriovascular malformation, adenocarcinoma, Henoch-Schönlein purpura, Pseudomembranous colitis

Gynecologic Disorders

Amenorrhea

Chief Complaint: Missed period.

History of Present Illness: Date of last menstrual period. Primary amenorrhea (absence of menses by age 16) or secondary amenorrhea (cessation of menses after previously normal menstruation). Age of menarche, menstrual regularity; age of breast development; sexual activity, possibility of pregnancy, pregnancy testing. Symptoms of pregnancy (nausea, breast tenderness).

Lifestyle changes, dieting, excessive exercise, drugs (marijuana), psychologic stress. Hot flushes (hypoestrogenism), galactorrhea (prolactinoma). Weight loss or gain, headaches, vision changes.

Past Medical History: History of dilation and curettage, postpartum infection (Asherman's syndrome), postpartum hemorrhage (Sheehan's syndrome); prior pregnancies.

Medications: Contraceptives, tricyclic antidepressants, digoxin, marijuana, chemotherapeutic agents.

Physical Examination

General Appearance: Secondary sexual characteristics, body habitus, obesity, deep voice (hyperandrogenism). Note whether the patient looks "ill" or well.

Vital Signs: Pulse (bradycardia), temperature (hypothermia, hypothyroidism), blood pressure, respirations.

Skin: Acne, hirsutism, temporal balding (hyperandrogenism, cool dry skin (hypothyroidism).

Eyes: Visual field defects, bitemporal hemianopsia (pituitary adenoma).

Neck: Thyroid enlargement or nodules.

Chest: Galactorrhea, impaired breast development, breast atrophy.

Heart: Bradycardia (hypothyroidism).

Abdomen: Abdominal striae (Cushing's syndrome).

Gyn: Pubic hair distribution, inguinal or labial masses, clitoromegaly, imperforate hymen, vaginal septum, vaginal atrophy, uterine enlargement, ovarian cysts or tumors.

Extremities: Tremor (hyperthyroidism).

Neurologic: Focal motor deficits.

Laboratory Evaluation: Pregnancy test, prolactin, TSH, free T_4. Progesterone challenge test.

Differential Diagnosis of Amenorrhea

Pregnancy
Hormonal contraception
Hypothalamic-related: Stress, ath-
   letics, eating disorder, obesity, drugs
   tumor
Pituitary-related: Hypopituitarism,
   tumor, infiltration, infarction
Ovarian-related: Dysgenesis, agenesis, ovarian failure

Outflow tract-related
   Imperforate hymen
   Transverse vaginal septum
   Agenesis of the vagina, cervix, uterus
   Uterine synechiae
Androgen excess
   Polycystic ovarian syndrome
   Adrenal tumor
   Adrenal hyperplasia
   Ovarian tumor
Other endocrine causes
   Thyroid disease
   Cushing syndrome

Abnormal Vaginal Bleeding

Chief Complaint: Abnormal vaginal bleeding.

History of Present Illness: Last menstrual period, number of soaked pads per day; menstrual regularity, age of menarche, duration and frequency of menses; passing of clots; postcoital or intermenstrual bleeding; abdominal pain, fever, lightheadedness; possibility of pregnancy, sexual activity, hormonal contraception.

Psychologic stress, weight changes, exercise. Changes in hair or skin texture.

Past Medical History: Obstetrical history. Thyroid, renal, or hepatic disease; coagulopathies, endometriosis, dental bleeding.

Family History: Coagulopathies, endocrine disorders.

Physical Examination

General Appearance: General body habitus, obesity. Note whether the patient looks "ill" or well.

Vital Signs: Assess hemodynamic stability, tachycardia, hypotension, orthostatic vitals; signs of shock.

Skin: Pallor, hirsutism, petechiae, skin texture; fine thinning hair (hypothyroidism).

Neck: Thyroid enlargement.

Breasts: Masses, galactorrhea.

Chest: Breath sounds.

Heart: Murmurs.

Gyn: Cervical motion tenderness, adnexal tenderness, uterine size, cervical lesions.

Laboratory Evaluation: CBC, platelets, beta-HCG, type and screen, cervix culture for N. gonorrhoeae, Chlamydia test, von Willebrand's screen, INR/PTT, bleeding time, pelvic ultrasound. Endometrial biopsy.

Differential Diagnosis of Abnormal Vaginal Bleeding: Chronic anovulation, pelvic inflammatory disease, cervicitis, pregnancy (ectopic pregnancy, spontaneous abortion, molar pregnancy). Hyperthyroidism, hypothyroidism, adrenal disease, diabetes mellitus. Hyperprolactinemia, polycystic ovary syndrome, oral contraceptives, medroxyprogesterone, anticoagulants, NSAIDs. Cervical polyps, uterine myoma endometriosis, retained tampon, trauma, Von Willebrand's disease.

Pelvic Pain and Ectopic Pregnancy

Chief Complaint: Pelvis pain.

History of Present Illness: Pelvic or abdominal pain (bilateral or unilateral), positive pregnancy test, missed menstrual period, abnormal vaginal bleeding (quantify). Date of last menstrual period. symptoms of pregnancy (breast tenderness, bloating); menstrual interval, duration, age of menarche, characteristics of pelvic pain; onset, duration, shoulder pain. Fever or vaginal discharge.

Past Medical History: Surgical history, sexually transmitted diseases, Chlamydia, gonorrhea, obstetrical history. Prior pelvic infection, endometriosis, prior ectopic pregnancy, pelvic tumor, intrauterine device.

Medications: Oral contraceptives.

Physical Examination

General Appearance: Moderate or severe distress. Note whether the patient looks "ill" or well.

Vital Signs: BP (orthostatic hypotension), pulse (tachycardia), respiratory rate (tachypnea), temperature (low fever).

Skin: Cold skin, pallor, delayed capillary refill.

Chest: Breath sounds.

Heart: Murmurs.

Abdomen: Cullen's sign (periumbilical darkening, intraabdominal bleeding), local then generalized tenderness, rebound tenderness.

Pelvic: Cervical discharge, cervical motion tenderness; Chadwick's sign (cervical cyanosis, pregnancy); Hegar's sign (softening of uterine isthmus, pregnancy); enlarged uterus, adnexal tenderness, cul-de-sac fullness.

Laboratory Evaluation: Quantitative beta-HCG, transvaginal ultrasound. Type and hold, Rh type, CBC, UA with micro; GC, chlamydia culture. Laparoscopy.

Differential Diagnosis of Pelvic Pain

Pregnancy-Related Causes: Ectopic pregnancy, spontaneous abortion, threatened abortion, incomplete abortion, intrauterine pregnancy with corpus luteum bleeding.

Gynecologic Disorders: Pelvic inflammatory disease, endometriosis, ovarian cyst hemorrhage or rupture, adnexal torsion, Mittelschmerz, primary dysmenorrhea, tumor.

Nonreproductive Causes of Pelvic Pain

Gastrointestinal: Appendicitis, inflammatory bowel disease, mesenteric adenitis, irritable bowel syndrome.

Urinary Tract: Urinary tract infection, renal calculus.

Neurologic Disorders

Headache

Chief Complaint: Headache

History of Present Illness: Quality of pain (dull, band-like, sharp, throbbing), location (retro-orbital, temporal, suboccipital, bilateral or unilateral); age of onset; time course of typical headache episode; rate of onset (gradual or sudden); time of day, effect of supine posture. Increasing frequency. Progression in severity. Does the headache interfere with normal activity or cause the child to stop playing? Awakening from sleep; analgesic use. "The worst headache ever" (subarachnoid hemorrhage).

Aura or Prodrome: Visual scotomata, blurred vision; nausea, vomiting, sensory disturbances.

Associated Symptoms: Numbness, weakness, diplopia, photophobia, fever, nasal discharge (sinusitis), neck stiffness (meningitis).

Aggravating or Relieving Factors: Relief by analgesics or sleep. Exacerbation by light or sounds, straining, exercising, or changing position. Exacerbation by foods (cheese), emotional upset, menses.

Past Medical History: Growth delay, development delay, allergies, past illnesses. Head injuries, motion sickness. Anxiety or depression

Medications: Dosage, frequency of use, and effect of medications. Birth control pills.

Family History: Migraine headaches in parents. Parental description of their headaches.

Social History: School absences. Stressful events. Emotional problems at home or in school. Cigarettes, alcohol, illegal drugs.

Review Systems: Changes in personality, memory, intellectual skills, vision, hearing, strength, gait, or balance. Postural lightheadedness, weakness, vertigo.

Physical Examination

General Appearance: Note whether the patient looks "ill" or well; interaction with parents; sad or withdrawn?

Vital Signs: BP (hypertension), pulse, temperature (fever), respiratory rate. Height, weight, head circumference; growth percentiles. Weight loss, lack of linear growth.

Skin: Pallor, petechiae, bruises. Alopecia, rashes, and painless oral ulcers. Café au lait spots in the axillae or inguinal areas (neurofibromatosis). Facial angiofibromas (adenoma sebaceum).

Head: Macrocephaly, cranial tenderness, temporal tenderness. Dilated scalp veins, frontal bossing. Sinuses tenderness (sinusitis) to percussion, temporal bruits (arteriovenous malformation).

Eyes: Downward deviation of the eyes ("sunset-ring" increased intracranial pressure), extraocular movements, pupil reactivity; papilledema, visual field deficits. Conjunctival injection, lacrimation (cluster headache).

Nose: Rhinorrhea (cluster headache).

Mouth: Tooth tenderness, gingivitis, pharyngeal erythema. Masseter muscle spasm, restricted jaw opening (TMJ dysfunction).

Neck: Rigidity, neck muscle tenderness.

Extremities: Absent femoral pulses, lower blood pressures in the legs (coarctation of the aorta).

Neurologic Examination: Mental status, cranial nerve function, motor strength, sensation, deep tendon reflexes. Disorientation, memory impairment, extraocular muscle dysfunction, spasticity, hyperreflexia, clonus, Babinski sign, ataxia, coordination.

Laboratory Evaluation: Electrolytes, ESR. CBC with differential, INR/PTT, MRI scan.

Recurrent and Chronic Headaches: Temporal Patterns	
Acute Recurrent Headache Migraine Cluster headache Acute sinusitis Hypertension Intermittent hydrocephalus Vascular malformation Subarachnoid hemorrhage Carbon monoxide poisoning **Chronic Nonprogressive Headache** Tension-type headache Chronic sinusitis Ocular disorder Dental abscess, temporomandibular joint syndrome Postlumbar puncture Posttraumatic headache	**Chronic Progressive Headache** Central nervous system infection Hydrocephalus Pseudotumor cerebri Brain tumor Vascular malformation Subdural hematoma Arnold-Chiari malformation Lead poisoning

Seizures, Spells and Unusual Movements

Chief Complaint: Seizure

History of Present Illness: Time of onset of seizure, duration, tonic-clonic movements, description of seizure, frequency of episodes, loss of consciousness. Past seizures, noncompliance with anticonvulsant medication. Aura before seizure (irritability, behavioral change, lethargy), incontinence of urine or feces, post-ictal weakness or paralysis, injuries. Can the patient tell when an episode will start? Warning signs, triggers for the spells (crying, anger, boredom, anxiety, fever, trauma). Does he speak during the spell? Does the child remember the spells afterward? What is the child like after the episode (confused, alert)? Can the child describe what happens?

Past Medical History: Illnesses, hospitalizations, previous functioning, rheumatic fever. Electroencephalograms, CT scans.

Medications: Antidepressants, stimulants, antiseizure medications.

Family History: Similar episodes in family, epilepsy, migraine, tics, tremors, Tourette syndrome, sleep disturbance. Rheumatic fever, streptococcal infection liver disease, metabolic disorders.

Physical Examination

General Appearance: Post-ictal lethargy. Note whether the patient looks well or ill. Observe the patient performing tasks (tying shoes, walking).

Vital Signs: Growth percentiles, BP (hypertension), pulse, respiratory rate, temperature (hyperpyrexia).

Skin: Café-au-lait spots, neurofibromas (Von Recklinghausen's disease). Unilateral port-wine facial nevus (Sturge-Weber syndrome); facial angiofibromas (adenoma sebaceum), hypopigmented ash leaf spots (tuberous sclerosis).

HEENT: Head trauma, pupil reactivity and equality, extraocular movements; papilledema, gum hyperplasia (phenytoin); tongue or buccal lacerations; neck rigidity.

Chest: Rhonchi, wheeze (aspiration).

Heart: Rhythm, murmurs.

Extremities: Cyanosis, fractures, trauma.

Perianal: Incontinence of urine or feces.

Neuro: Dysarthria, visual field deficits, cranial nerve palsies, sensory deficits, focal weakness (Todd's paralysis), Babinski's sign, developmental delay.

Laboratory Evaluation: Glucose, electrolytes, CBC, urine toxicology, anticonvulsant levels, RPR/VDRL, EEG, MRI, lumbar puncture.

Differential Diagnosis of Seizures, Spells, and Unusual Movements

Epilepsy	Choreoathetosis
Movement disorders	Benign
Tics	Familial
Myoclonic syndromes	Paroxysmal
Sleep	Sydenham chorea
Benign	Huntington chorea
Hyperexplexia (exaggerated startle response)	Drugs
	Behavioral/Psychiatric Disorders
Myoclonus-opsoclonus	**Pseudoseizures**
Shuddering spells	**Automatisms**
Dystonia	**Dyscontrol syndrome**
Torsion	**Attention-deficit hyperactivity disorder**
Transient torticollis	**Benign paroxysmal vertigo**
Sandifer syndrome	**Migraine**
Drugs	**Parasomnias**
Dyskinesias	**Syncope**
Metabolic/genetic	**Breathholding spells**
Reflex dystrophy	
Nocturnal	
Physiologic	

Apnea

Chief Complaint: Apnea.

History of Present Illness: Length of pause in respiration. Change in skin color (cyanosis, pallor), hypotonia or hypertonia, resuscitative efforts (rescue breaths, chest compressions). Stridor, wheezing, body position during the event, state of consciousness before, during and after the event. Unusual movements, incontinence, postictal confusional state. Regurgitation after feedings. Vomitus in oral cavity during the event.

Loud snoring, nocturnal enuresis, excessive daytime sleepiness; prior acute life-threatening events (ALTEs). Medications accessible to the child in the home.

Past Medical History: Abnormal growth, developmental delay, asthma.

Perinatal History: Prenatal exposure to infectious agents, maternal exposure to opioids, difficulties during labor and delivery. Respiratory difficulties after birth.

Immunizations: Pertussis.

Family History: Genetic or metabolic disorders, mental retardation, consanguinity, fetal loss, neonatal death, sudden infant death syndrome, elicit drugs, alcohol.

Social history: Physical abuse, previous involvement of the family with child protective services.

Physical Examination

General Appearance: Septic appearance, level of consciousness.

Vital Signs: Length, weight, head circumference percentiles. Pulse, blood pressure, respirations, temperature.

Skin: Cool, mottled extremities; delayed capillary refill, bruises, scars.

Nose: Nasal flaring, nasal secretions, mucosal erythema, obstruction, septal deviation or polyps.

Mouth: Structure of the lips, tongue, palate; tonsillar lesions, masses.

Neck: Masses, enlarged lymph nodes, enlarged thyroid.

Chest: Increased respiratory effort, intercostal retractions, barrel chest. Irregular respirations, periodic breathing, prolonged pauses in respiration, stridor. Grunting, wheezing, crackles.

Heart: Rate and rhythm, S1, S2, murmurs. Preductal and postductal pulse delay (right arm and leg pulse comparison).

Abdomen: Hepatomegaly, nephromegaly.

Extremities: Dependent edema, digital clubbing.

Neurologic: Mental status, muscle tone, strength. Cranial nerve function, gag reflex.

Laboratory Evaluation: Glucose, electrolytes, BUN, creatinine, calcium, magnesium, CBC, ECG, O_2 saturation.

Differential Diagnosis of Apnea

Central Nervous System
  Dandy-Walker malformation
  Arnold-Chiari malformation
  Seizures
  Hypotonia, weakness
  Ondine's curse
Metabolic/Toxic
  Hypoglycemia
  Hypocalcemia
  Hyponatremia
  Acidosis
  Hypomagnesemia
  Opioids
  Medium-chain acyl-CoA
  dehydrogenase deficiency
Upper Airway
  Craniofacial syndromes
  Laryngomalacia
  Rhinitis
  Choanal stenosis/atresia
  Croup

Upper Airway (continued)
  Adenotonsillar hypertrophy
  Epiglottitis
  Post-extubation
  Vocal cord paralysis
  Anaphylaxis
Lower Airway
  Pneumonia
  Bronchiolitis
  Pertussis
Cardiovascular
  Structural disease
  Dysrhythmia
Gastrointestinal
  Gastroesophageal reflux
Miscellaneous
  Sepsis
  Meningitis
  Munchausen syndrome by proxy

Delirium, Coma and Confusion

Chief Complaint: Confusion.

History of Present Illness: Level of consciousness, obtundation (awake but not alert), stupor (unconscious but awakable with vigorous stimulation), coma (cannot be awakened). Confusion, impaired concentration, agitation. Fever, headache. Activity and symptoms prior to onset.

Past Medical History: Suicide attempts or depression, epilepsy (post-ictal state).

Medications: Insulin, narcotics, drugs, anticholinergics.

Physical Examination

General Appearance: Incoherent speech, lethargy, somnolence. Dehydration, septic appearance. Note whether the patient looks "ill" or well.

Vital Signs: BP (hypertensive encephalopathy), pulse, temperature (fever), respiratory rate.

Skin: Cyanosis, jaundice, delayed capillary refill, petechia, splinter hemorrhages; injection site fat atrophy (diabetes).

Head: Skull tenderness, lacerations, ptosis, facial weakness. Battle's sign (ecchymosis over mastoid process), raccoon sign (periorbital ecchymosis, skull fracture), hemotympanum (basal skull fracture).

Eyes: Pupil size and reactivity, extraocular movements, papilledema.

Mouth: Tongue or cheek lacerations; atrophic tongue, glossitis (B12 deficiency).

Neck: Neck rigidity, masses.

Chest: Breathing pattern (Cheyne-Stokes hyperventilation), crackles, wheezes.

Heart: Rhythm, murmurs, gallops.

Abdomen: Hepatomegaly, splenomegaly, masses.

Neuro: Strength, cranial nerves 2-12, mini-mental status exam; orientation to person, place, time, recent events; Babinski's sign, primitive reflexes (snout, suck, glabella, palmomental grasp).

Laboratory Evaluation: Glucose, electrolytes, BUN, creatinine, O_2 saturation, liver function tests. CT/MRI, urine toxicology screen.

Differential Diagnosis of Delirium: Hypoxia, meningitis, encephalitis, systemic infection, electrolyte imbalance, hyperglycemia, hypoglycemia (insulin overdose), drug intoxication, stroke, intracranial hemorrhage, seizure; dehydration, head trauma, uremia, vitamin B12 deficiency, ketoacidosis, factitious coma.

Renal and Endocrinologic Disorders

Polyuria, Enuresis and Urinary Frequency

Chief Complaint: Excessive urination.

History of Present Illness: Time of onset of excessive urination. Constant daytime thirst or waking at night to drink. Poor urinary stream, persistent dribbling of urine; straining to urinate. Excessive fluid intake, dysuria, recurrent urinary tract infections; urgency, daytime and nighttime enuresis, fever. Gait disturbances, history of lumbar puncture, spinal cord injury. Lower extremity weakness; back pain, leg pain. Use of harsh soaps for bathing. Feeding schedule, overfeeding, growth pattern, dehydration. Vomiting, constipation. Abdominal and perineal pain, constipation, encopresis

Past Medical History: Urinary tract infections, diabetes, renal disease.

Social History: History of foreign body insertion or sexual abuse.

Family History: Family members with polydipsia, polyuria; early infant deaths, infants with poor growth or dehydration; genitourinary disorders. Parental age of toilet training.

Physical Examination

General Appearance: Signs of dehydration, septic appearance.

Vital Signs: Blood pressure (hypertension), pulse (tachycardia), temperature, respirations. Growth percentiles, growth failure.

Chest: Breath sounds.

Heart: Murmurs, third heart sound.

Abdomen: Masses, palpable bladder. Perineal excoriation; lumbosacral midline defects, sacral hairy patch, sacral hyperpigmentation, sacral dimple or sinus tract, hemangiomas.

Rectal Examination: Rectal sphincter laxity, anal reflex (sacral nerve function).

Extremities: Asymmetric gluteal cleft, gluteal lipoma, gluteal wasting.

Neurologic Examination: Deep tendon reflexes, muscle strength in the legs and feet. Perineal sensation, gait disturbance.

Differential Diagnosis of Polyuria

Water Diuresis
Primary polydipsia
Diabetes insipidus
Obstruction by posterior urethral valves, uteropelvic junction obstruction, ectopic ureter, nephrolithiasis
Renal infarction secondary to sickle-cell disease
Chronic pyelonephritis
Solute Diuresis: Glucose, urea, mannitol, sodium chloride, mineralocorticoid deficiency or excess, alkali ingestion

Differential Diagnosis of Enuresis and Urinary Frequency	
Infection	Diabetes insipidus
Uteropelvic junction obstruction	Wilms tumor
Obstructive ectopic ureter	Neuroblastoma
Posterior urethral valves	Pelvic tumors
Nephrolithiasis	Fecal impaction
Diabetes mellitus	

Hematuria

Chief Complaint: Blood in urine.

History of Present Illness: Color of urine, duration and timing of hematuria. Frequency, dysuria, suprapubic pain, flank pain (renal colic), abdominal or perineal pain, fever, menstruation.

Foley catheterization, stone passage, tissue passage in urine, joint pain.

Strenuous exercise, dehydration, recent trauma. Rashes, arthritis (systemic lupus erythematosus, Henoch-Schönlein purpura). Bloody diarrhea (hemolytic-uremic syndrome), hepatitis B or C exposure.

Causes of Red Urine: Pyridium, phenytoin, ibuprofen, cascara laxatives, rifampin, berries, flava beans, food coloring, rhubarb, beets, hemoglobinuria, myoglobinuria.

Past Medical History: Recent sore throat (group A streptococcus), streptococcal skin infection (glomerulonephritis). Recent or recurrent upper respiratory illness (adenovirus).

Medications Associated with Hematuria: Warfarin, aspirin, ibuprofen, naproxen, phenobarbital, phenytoin, cyclophosphamide.

Perinatal History: Birth asphyxia, umbilical catheterization.

Family History: Hematuria, renal disease, sickle cell anemia, bleeding disorders, hemophilia, deafness (Alport's syndrome), hypertension.

Social History: Occupational exposure to toxins.

Physical Examination

General Appearance: Signs of dehydration. Note whether the patient looks "ill" or well.

Vital Signs: Hypertension (acute renal failure, acute glomerulonephritis), fever, respiratory rate, pulse.

Skin: Pallor, malar rash, discoid rash (systemic lupus erythematosus); ecchymoses, petechiae (Henoch-Schönlein purpura).

Face: Periorbital edema (nephritis, nephrotic syndrome).

Eyes: Lens dislocation, dot-and-fleck retinopathy (Alport's syndrome).

Throat: Pharyngitis.

Chest: Breath sounds.

Heart: Rhythm, murmurs, gallops.

Abdomen: Masses, nephromegaly (Wilms' tumor, polycystic kidney disease, hydronephrosis), abdominal bruits, suprapubic tenderness.

Back: Costovertebral angle tenderness (renal calculus, pyelonephritis).

Genitourinary: Discharge, foreign body, trauma, meatal stenosis.

Extremities: Peripheral edema (nephrotic syndrome), joint swelling, joint tenderness (rheumatic fever), unequal peripheral pulses (aortic coarctation).

Laboratory Evaluation: Urinalysis with microscopic, urine culture; creatinine, BUN, CBC; sickle cell screen; urine calcium-to-creatinine ratio, INR/PTT. Urinalysis of first-degree relatives (Alport's syndrome or benign familial hematuria), renal ultrasonography.

Specific Laboratory Evaluation: Complement levels, anti-streptolysin-O and anti-DNAse B (poststreptococcal glomerulonephritis), antinuclear antibody, audiogram (Alport's syndrome), antiglomerular basement membrane antibodies (Goodpasture's syndrome), antineutrophil cytoplasmic antibodies, purified protein derivative (PPD).

Advanced Laboratory Evaluation: Voiding cystourethrogram, intravenous pyelography, CT scan, MRI scan, renal scan, renal biopsy.

Differential Diagnosis of Microscopic Hematuria

Glomerular Diseases

Benign familial or sporadic hematuria (thin membrane nephropathy)	Membranoproliferative glomerulo-nephritis
Acute postinfectious glomerulonephritis	Systemic lupus erythematosus
Hemolytic-uremic syndrome	Henoch-Schönlein nephritis
IgA nephropathy (Berger's disease)	Polyarteritis
Alport's syndrome (familial nephritis)	Hepatitis-associated glomerulonephritis
Focal segmental glomerulonephritis	

Nonglomerular Diseases

Strenuous exercise	Leukemia
Dehydration	Coagulopathy
Fever	Anatomical abnormalities
Menstruation	Hydronephrosis
Foreign body in urethra or bladder	Ureteropelvic junction obstruction
Urinary tract infection: bacterial, adenovirus, tuberculosis	Cystic kidneys
Hypercalciuria	Polycystic kidney disease
Urolithiasis	Medullary cystic disease
Sickle cell trait or disease	Vascular malformations
Trauma	Arteriovenous fistula
Drugs and toxins	Renal vein thrombosis
Masturbation	Nutcracker syndrome
Tumors	Papillary necrosis
Wilms' tumor	Parenchymal infarction
Tuberous sclerosis	Munchausen syndrome-by-proxy
Renal or bladder cancer	

Proteinuria

Chief Complaint: Proteinuria.

History of Present Illness: Protein of 1+ (30 mg/dL) on a urine dipstick. Protein above 4 mg/m^2/hour in a timed 12- to 24-hour urine collection (significant proteinuria). Prior proteinuria, hypertension, edema; short stature, hearing deficits.

Past Medical History: Renal disease, heart disease, arthralgias.

Medications: Chemotherapy agents.

Family History: Renal disease, deafness.

Physical Examination
General Appearance: Signs of dehydration. Note whether the patient looks "ill" or well.
Vital Signs: Temperature (fever).
Ears: Dysmorphic pinnas.
Skin: Café-au-lait spots, hypopigmented macules, rash.
Extremities: Joint tenderness, joint swelling.
Laboratory Evaluation: Urinalysis for spot protein/creatinine ratio. Recumbent and ambulating urinalyses. CBC, electrolytes, BUN, creatinine, total protein, albumin, cholesterol, antistreptolysin-O titer (ASO), antinuclear antibody, complement levels. Renal ultrasound, voiding cystourethrogram.

Differential Diagnosis of Proteinuria

Functional/Transient (<2+ on urine dipstick)
Fever
Strenuous exercise
Cold exposure
Congestive heart failure
Seizures
Emotional stress

Isolated Proteinuria
Orthostatic proteinuria (60% of cases)
Persistent asymptomatic proteinuria

Glomerular Disease
Minimal change nephrotic syndrome
Glomerulonephritis
  Postinfectious
  Membranoproliferative
  Membranous
  IgA nephropathy
  Henoch-Schönlein purpura
  Systemic lupus erythematosus
  Hereditary nephritis

Tubulointerstitial Disease
Reflux nephropathy
Interstitial nephritis
Hypokalemic nephropathy
Cystinosis
Fanconi's syndrome
Tyrosinemia

Lowe syndrome
Tubular toxins
  Drugs (eg, aminoglycosides and penicillins)
  Heavy metals
Ischemic tubular injury

Swelling and Edema

Chief Complaint: Swollen ankles.

History of Present Illness: Duration of edema; distribution (localized or generalized); intermittent or persistent swelling, pain, redness. Renal disease; shortness of breath, malnutrition, chronic diarrhea (protein losing enteropathy), allergies. Periorbital edema, ankle edema, weight gain.

Poor exercise tolerance, fatigue, inability to keep up with other children. Poor feeding, fussiness, restlessness. Bloody urine (smoky or red), decreased urine output, jaundice. Poor protein intake (Kwashiorkor), dietary history.

Past Medical History: Menstrual cycle, sexual activity, premenstrual bloating, pregnancy, rash.

Medications: Over-the-counter drugs, diuretics, oral contraceptives, anti-hypertensives, estrogen, lithium.

Allergies: Allergic reactions to foods (cow's milk).

Family History: Lupus erythematosus, cystic fibrosis, renal disease, Alport syndrome, hereditary angioedema, deafness.

Social History: Exposure to toxins, illicit drugs, alcohol, chemicals.

Physical Examination

General Appearance: Respiratory distress, pallor. Note whether the patient looks "ill" or well.

Vitals: BP (upright and supine), pulse (tachycardia), temperature, respiratory rate (tachypnea). Growth percentiles, poor weight gain. Decreased urine output.

Skin: Xanthomata, spider angiomata, cyanosis. Rash, insect bite puncta, erythema.

HEENT: Periorbital edema. Conjunctival injection, scleral icterus, nasal polyps, sinus tenderness, pharyngitis.

Chest: Breath sounds, crackles, dullness to percussion.

Heart: Displacement of point of maximal impulse; silent precordium, S3 gallop, friction rub, murmur.

Abdomen: Distention, bruits, hepatomegaly, splenomegaly, shifting dullness.

Extremities: Pitting or non-pitting edema (graded 1 to 4+), erythema, pulses, clubbing.

Laboratory Evaluation: Electrolytes, liver function tests, triglycerides, albumin, CBC, chest x-ray, urine protein.

Differential Diagnosis of Edema

Increased Hydrostatic Pressure
Congestive heart failure
Pericarditis
Superior vena cava syndrome
Arteriovenous fistula
Venous thrombosis
Lymphatic obstruction by tumors
Syndrome of inappropriate ADH secretion
Steroids
Excessive Iatrogenic fluid administration

Increased Capillary Permeability
Rocky Mountain spotted fever
Stevens-Johnson syndrome

Decreased Oncotic Pressure (Hypoproteinemia)
Nephrotic syndrome
Liver disease (alpha$_1$-antitrypsin deficiency, infectious hepatitis)
Cirrhosis
Galactosemia
Kwashiorkor
Marasmus
Cystic fibrosis
Inflammatory bowel disease
Protein-losing enteropathy (cow's milk allergy)
Intestinal lymphangiectasia
Celiac disease
Bezoar
Infection (Giardia sp.)
Pancreatic pseudocyst
Severe anemia
Zinc deficiency

Diabetic Ketoacidosis

Chief Complaint: Malaise.

History of Present Illness: Initial glucose level, ketones, anion gap. Duration of polyuria, polyphagia, polydipsia, lethargy, dyspnea, weight loss; noncompliance with insulin; blurred vision, infection, dehydration, abdominal pain (appendicitis). Cough, fever, chills, ear pain (otitis media), dysuria (urinary tract infection).

Factors that May Precipitate Diabetic Ketoacidosis. New onset of diabetes, noncompliance with insulin, infection, pancreatitis, myocardial infarction, stress, trauma, pregnancy.

Past Medical History: Age of onset of diabetes; renal disease, infections, hospitalization.

Physical Examination

General Appearance: Somnolence, Kussmaul respirations (deep sighing breathing), dehydration. Note whether the patient looks "toxic" or well.

Vital Signs: BP (hypotension), pulse (tachycardia), temperature (fever, hypothermia), respiratory rate (tachypnea).

Skin: Decreased skin turgor, delayed capillary refill, intertriginous candidiasis, erythrasma, localized fat atrophy (insulin injections).

Eyes: Diabetic retinopathy (neovascularization, hemorrhages), decreased visual acuity.

Mouth: Acetone breath odor (musty, apple odor), dry mucous membranes (dehydration).

Ears: Tympanic membrane erythema (otitis media).

Chest: Rales, rhonchi (pneumonia).

Heart: Murmurs.

Abdomen: Hypoactive bowel sounds (ileus), right lower quadrant tenderness (appendicitis), suprapubic tenderness (cystitis), costovertebral angle tenderness (pyelonephritis).

Extremities: Abscesses, cellulitis.

Neurologic: Confusion, hyporeflexia.

Laboratory Evaluation: Glucose, sodium, potassium, bicarbonate, chloride, BUN, creatinine, anion gap, phosphate, CBC, serum ketones; UA (proteinuria, ketones). Chest x-ray.

Differential Diagnosis

   Ketosis-causing Conditions: Alcoholic ketoacidosis or starvation.

   Acidosis-causing Conditions

      Increased Anion Gap Acidoses: Lactic acidosis, uremia, salicylate or methanol poisoning.

      Non-Anion Gap Acidoses: Diarrhea, renal tubular acidosis.

Diagnostic Criteria for DKA. Glucose ≥ 250, pH <7.3, bicarbonate <15, ketone positive $>1:2$ dilutions.

Dermatologic, Hematologic and Rheumatologic Disorders

Rash

Chief Complaint: Rash.

History of Present Illness: Time of rash onset, location, pattern of spread (chest to extremities). Location where the rash first appeared; what it resembled; what symptoms were associated with it; what treatments have been tried. Fever, malaise, headache; conjunctivitis, coryza, cough. Exposure to persons with rash, prior history of chicken pox. Sore throat, joint pain, abdominal pain. Exposure to allergens or irritants. Sun exposure, cold, psychologic stress.

Past Medical History: Prior rashes, asthma, allergic rhinitis, urticaria, eczema, diabetes, hospitalizations, surgery.

Medications: Prescription and nonprescription, drug reactions.

Family History: Similar problems among family members.

Immunizations: Vaccination status, measles, mumps, rubella.

Social History: Drugs, alcohol, home situation.

Physical Examination

General Appearance: Respiratory distress, toxic appearance.

Vital Signs: Temperature, pulse, blood pressure, respirations.

Skin: Complete skin examination, including the nails and mucous membranes. Color or surface changes, texture changes, warmth. Distribution of skin lesions (face, trunk, extremities), shape of the lesions, arrangement of several lesions (annular, serpiginous, dermatomal); color of the lesions, dominant hue and the color pattern, surface characteristics (scaly, verrucous), erythema, papules, induration, flat, macules, vesicles, ulceration, margin character, lichenification, excoriations, crusting.

Eyes: Conjunctival erythema.

Ears: Tympanic membranes.

Mouth: Soft palate macules; buccal mucosa lesions.

Throat: Pharyngeal erythema.

Lymph Nodes: Cervical, axillary, inguinal lymphadenopathy.

Chest: Rhonchi, crackles , wheezing.

Heart: Murmurs.

Abdomen: Tenderness, masses, hepatosplenomegaly.

Extremities: Rash on hands, feet, palms, soles; joint swelling, joint tenderness.

Differential Diagnosis: Varicella, rubella, measles, scarlet fever, eczema, dermatitis, rocky mountain spotted fever, drug eruption, Kawasaki's disease.

Laboratory Diagnosis: Virus isolation or antigen detection (blood, nasopharynx, conjunctiva, urine). Acute and convalescent antibody titers.

Bruising and Bleeding

Chief Complaint: Bruising

History of Present Illness: Time of onset of bruising; trauma, spontaneous ecchymoses, petechiae; bleeding gums, bleeding into joints, epistaxis, hematemesis, melena. Bone pain, joint pain, abdominal pain. Is the bleeding lifelong or of recent onset? Hematuria, extensive bleeding with trauma. Weight loss, fever, pallor, jaundice, recurring infections.

Past Medical History: Oozing from the umbilical stump after birth, bleeding at injection sites. Prolonged bleeding after minor surgery (circumcision) or after loss of primary teeth.

Family History: Bleeding disorders, anticoagulant use, availability of rodenticides or antiplatelet drugs (eg, aspirin or other nonsteroidals) in the home. Child abuse.

Social History: History of child abuse, family stress.

Physical Examination

General Appearance: Ill-appearance.

Vital Signs: Tachypnea, tachycardia, fever, blood pressure (orthostatic changes), cachexia.

Skin: Appearance and distribution of petechiae (color, size, shape, diffuse, symmetrical), ecchymotic patterns (eg, belt buckle shape, doubled-over phone cord); folliculitis (neutropenia). Hyperextensible skin (Ehlers-Danlos syndrome). Partial albinism (Hermansky-Pudlak syndrome). Palpable purpura on legs (vasculitis, Henoch-Schönlein purpura).

Lymph Nodes: Cervical or axillary lymphadenopathy

Eyes: Conjunctival pallor, erythema.

Nose: Epistaxis, nasal eschar.

Mouth: Gingivitis, mucous membrane bleeding, oozing from gums, oral petechiae.

Chest: Wheezing, rhonchi.

Heart: Murmurs.

Abdomen: Hepatomegaly, splenomegaly, nephromegaly.

Rectal: Stool occult blood.

Extremities: Muscle hematomas; anomalies of the radius bone (thrombocytopenia absent radius [TAR] syndrome). Bone tenderness, joint tenderness, hemarthroses; hypermobile joints (Ehlers-Danlos syndrome.

Past Testing: X-ray studies, endoscopy.

Differential Diagnosis of Bruising and Bleeding	
Hemolytic uremic syndrome	Takayasu arteritis
Thrombotic thrombocytopenic purpura	Polyarteritis nodosa
Uremia	Kawasaki syndrome
Paraproteinemia	Henoch-Schönlein purpura
Myelodysplastic syndrome	Leukocytoclastic ("hypersensitivity")
Phenytoin, valproic acid, quinidine,	vasculitis
heparin	Wegener granulomatosis
Afibrinogenemia/dysfibrinogenemia	Churg-Strauss syndrome
Clotting factor deficiencies (hemophilia	Essential cryoglobulinemia
A, B, Christmas disease)	Systemic lupus erythematosus
Von Willebrand disease	Juvenile rheumatoid arthritis
Vitamin K deficiency	Mixed connective tissue disease
Hemorrhagic disease of the newborn	Dermatomyositis, scleroderma
Trauma	Bacterial or viral infection, spirochetal
Vasculitis	infection, rickettsial infection
Giant cell (temporal) arteritis	Malignancy

Kawasaki Disease

Chief Complaint: Fever.

History of Present Illness: Fever of unknown cause, lasting 5 days or more; irritability, chest pain. Eye redness. Redness, dryness or fissuring of lips, strawberry tongue. Diarrhea, vomiting, abdominal pain, arthritis/arthralgias. Absence of cough, rhinorrhea, vomiting.

Physical Examination

General Appearance: Ill appearance, irritable.

Vital Signs: Pulse (tachycardia), blood pressure (hypotension), respirations, temperature (fever).

Skin: Diffuse polymorphous rash (macules, bullae, erythematous exanthem) of the trunk; morbilliform or scarlatiniform rash.

Eyes: Bilateral conjunctival congestion (dilated blood vessels without purulent discharge), erythema, conjunctival suffusion, uveitis.

Mouth: Erythema of lips, fissures of lips; swollen, erythematous tongue. Diffuse injection of oral and pharyngeal mucosa.

Lymph Nodes: Cervical lymphadenopathy.

Chest: Breath sounds.

Heart: Murmur, gallop rhythm, distant heart sounds.

Abdomen: Tenderness, hepatomegaly, splenomegaly.

Extremities: Edema, erythema of the hands and feet; warm, red, swollen hands and feet. Joint swelling, joint tenderness. Desquamation of the fingers or toes, usually around nails and spreading over palms and soles (late).

Laboratory Evaluation: CBC with differential, platelet count, electrolytes, liver function tests, ESR, CRP, throat culture, antistreptolysin-O titer, blood cultures.

Urinalysis: Proteinuria, increase of leukocytes in urine sediment (sterile pyuria)

ECG: Prolonged PR, QT intervals, abnormal Q wave, low voltage, ST-T changes, arrhythmias.

CXR: Cardiomegaly

Echocardiography: Pericardial effusion, coronary aneurysm, myocardial infarction.

Differential Diagnosis: Scarlet fever (no hand, foot, or conjunctival involvement), Stevens-Johnson syndrome (mouth sores, cutaneous bullae, crusts), measles (rash occurs after fever peaks and begins on head/scalp), toxic shock syndrome, viral syndrome, drug reaction.

Behavioral Disorders and Trauma

Failure to Thrive

Chief Complaint: Inadequate growth.

History of Present Illness: Weight loss, change in appetite, vomiting, abdominal pain, diarrhea, fever. Date when the parents became concerned about the problem, previous hospitalizations. Polyuria, polydipsia; jaundice; cough.

Nutritional History: Appropriate caloric intake, 24-hour diet recall; dietary calendar; types and amounts of food offered. Proper formula preparation. Parental dietary restrictions (low fat).

Past Medical History: Excessive crying, feeding problems. Poor suck and swallow, fatigue during feeding. Unexplained injuries.

Developmental History: Developmental delay, loss of developmental milestones.

Perinatal History: Delayed intrauterine growth, maternal illness, medications or drugs (tobacco, alcohol). Birth weight, perinatal jaundice, feeding difficulties.

Family History: Short stature, parental heights and the ages at which the parents achieved puberty. Siblings with poor growth. Deaths in siblings or relatives during early childhood (metabolic or immunologic disorders).

Social History: Parental HIV-risk behavior (bisexual exposure, intravenous drug abuse, blood transfusions). Parental histories of neglect or abuse in childhood; current stress within the family, financial difficulties, marital discord.

Historical Findings in Failure to Thrive	
Poor Caloric Intake	Diarrhea, dysentery, fever
Breast-feeding mismanagement	Inflammatory bowel disease
Lactation failure	Radiation, chemotherapy
Improper formula preparation	Hypogeusia, anorexia
Maternal stress, poor diet, illness	Recurrent infections
Eating disorders	Rash, arthritis, weakness
Aberrant parental nutritional beliefs	Jaundice
Food faddism	Polyuria, polydipsia, polyphagia
Diaphoresis or fatigue while eating	Irritability, constipation
Poor suck, swallow	Mental retardation, swallowing difficulties
Vomiting, hyperkinesis	
Bilious vomiting	Intrauterine growth delay
Recurrent pneumonias, steatorrhea	

Physical Examination

General Appearance: Cachexia, dehydration. Note whether the patient looks "ill," well, or malnourished. Observation of parent-child interaction; affection, warmth. Passive or withdrawn behavior. Decreased vocalization, expressionless facies; increased hand and finger activities (thumb sucking), infantile posture; motor inactivity (congenital encephalopathy or rubella).

Developmental Examination: Delayed abilities for age on developmental screening test.

Vital Signs: Pulse (bradycardia), BP, respiratory rate, temperature (hypothermia). Weight, length, and head circumference; short stature, growth percentiles.

Skin: Pallor, jaundice, skin laxity, rash.

Lymph Nodes: Cervical or supraclavicular lymphadenopathy.

Head: Temporal wasting, congenital malformations.

Eyes: Cataracts (rubella), icterus, dry conjunctiva.

Mouth: Dental erosions, oropharyngeal lesions, cheilosis (cobalamin deficiency), glossitis (Pellagra).

Neck: Thyromegaly.

Chest: Barrel shaped chest, rhonchi.

Heart: Displaced point of maximal impulse, patent ductus arteriosus murmur, aortic stenosis murmur.

Abdomen: Protuberant abdomen, decreased bowel sounds (malabsorption, obstructive uropathy), tenderness. Periumbilical adenopathy. Masses (pyloric stenosis or obstructive uropathy), hepatomegaly (galactosemia), splenomegaly.

Extremities: Edema, muscle wasting.

Neuro: Decreased peripheral sensation.

Rectal: Occult blood, masses.

Genitalia: Hypospadias (obstructive uropathy).

Physical Examination Findings in Growth Deficiency

Micrognathia, cleft lip and palate	Short stature
Poor suck, swallow	Cachexia, mass
Hyperkinesis	Rash, joint erythema, tenderness, weakness
Bulging fontanelle, papilledema	
Nystagmus, ataxia	Jaundice, hepatomegaly
Abdominal distension	Ambiguous genitalia, masculinization
Fever	
Clubbing	Irritability
Perianal skin tags	

Laboratory Evaluation: CBC, electrolytes, protein, albumin, transferrin, thyroid studies, liver function tests.

Differential Diagnosis of Failure to Thrive

Poor Caloric Intake
  Breast-feeding mismanagement
  Lactation failure
  Maternal stress, poor diet, illness
  Eating disorders (older children)
  Aberrant parental nutritional beliefs
  Food faddism
  Improper formula preparation
  Micrognathia, cleft lip, cleft palate
  Cardiopulmonary disease
  Hypotonia, CNS disease
  Diencephalic syndrome

Poor Caloric Retention
  Increased intracranial pressure
  Labyrinthine disorders
  Esophageal obstruction, gastroesophageal reflux, preampullary obstruction
  Intestinal obstruction, volvulus, Hirschsprung disease
  Metabolic disorders

Poor Caloric Digestion/Assimilation/Absorption
  Cystic fibrosis
  Shwachman-Diamond syndrome
  Fat malabsorption
  Enteric infections
  Infection
  Inflammatory bowel disease
  Cancer treatment
  Gluten-sensitive enteropathy
  Carbohydrate malabsorption
  Intestinal lymphangiectasia
  Zinc deficiency

Increased Caloric Demands
  Chronic infection
  HIV infection
  Malignancies
  Autoimmune disorders
  Chronic renal disease
  Chronic liver disease
  Diabetes mellitus
  Adrenal hyperplasia
  Hypercalcemia
  Hypothyroidism
  Metabolic errors

Miscellaneous
  CNS impairment
  Prenatal growth failure
  Short stature
  Lagging-down
  Normal thinness

Developmental Delay

Chief Complaint: Delayed development.
Developmental History: Age when parents first became concerned about delayed development. Rate and pattern of acquisition of skills; developmental regressions. Parents' description of the child's current skills. How does he move around? How does he use his hands? How does he let you know what he wants? What does he understand of what you say? What can you tell him to do? What does he like to play with? How does he play with toys? How does he interact with other children?
Behavior in early infancy (quality of alertness, responsiveness). Developmental quotient (DQ): Developmental age divided by the child's chronologic age x

100. Vision and hearing deficits.

Perinatal History: In utero exposure to toxins or teratogens, maternal illness or trauma, complications of pregnancy. Quality of fetal movement, poor fetal weight gain (placental dysfunction). Apgar scores, neonatal seizures, poor feeding, poor muscle tone at birth. Growth parameters at birth, head circumference.

Past Medical History: Illnesses, poor feeding, vomiting, failure to thrive. Weak sucking and swallowing, excessive drooling.

Medications: Anticonvulsants, stimulants.

Family History: Illnesses, hearing impairment, mental retardation, mental illness, language problems, learning disabilities, dyslexia, consanguinity.

Social History: Home situation, toxin exposure, lead exposure.

Physical Examination

Observation: Facial expressions, eye contact, social, interaction with caretakers and examiner. Chronically ill, wasted, malnourished appearance, lethargic/fatigued.

Vital Signs: Respirations, pulse, blood pressure, temperature. Height, weight, head circumference, growth percentiles.

Skin: Café au lait spots, hypopigmented macules (neurofibromatosis), hemangiomas, telangiectasias, axillary freckling. Cyanosis, jaundice, pallor, skin turgor.

Head: Frontal bossing, low anterior hairline; head size, shape, circumference, microcephaly, macrocephaly, asymmetry, cephalohematoma; short palpebral fissure, flattened mid-face (fetal alcohol syndrome), chin shape (prominent or small).

Eyes: Size, shape, and distance between the eyes (small palpebral fissures, hypotelorism, hypertelorism, upslanting or downslanting palpebral fissures). Retinopathy, cataracts, corneal clouding, visual acuity. Lens dislocation, corneal clouding, strabismus.

Ears: Size and placement of the pinnae (low-set, posteriorly rotated, cupped, small, prominent). Tympanic membranes, hearing.

Nose: Broad nasal bridge, short nose, anteverted nares.

Mouth: Hypoplastic philtrum. Lip thinness, downturned corners, fissures, cleft, teeth (caries, discoloration), mucus membrane color and moisture.

Lymph Nodes: Location, size, tenderness, mobility, consistency.

Neck: Position, mobility, swelling, thyroid nodules.

Lungs: Breathing rate, depth, chest expansion, crackles.

Heart: Location and intensity of apical impulse, murmurs.

Abdomen: Contour, bowel sounds, tenderness, tympany; hepatomegaly, splenomegaly, masses.

Genitalia: Ambiguous genitalia (hypogonadism).

Extremities: Posture, gait, stance, asymmetry of movement. Edema, clinodactyly, syndactyly, nail deformities, palmar or plantar simian crease.

Neurological Examination: Behavior, level of consciousness, intelligence, emotional status. Equilibrium reactions (slowly tilting and observing for compensatory movement). Protective reactions (displacing to the side and observing for arm extension by 7 to 8 months).

Motor System: Gait, muscle tone, muscle strength (graded 0 to 5), deep tenon reflexes.

Primitive Reflexes: Palmar grasp, Moro, asymmetric tonic neck reflexes.

Signs of Cerebral Palsy: Fisting with adducted thumbs, hyperextension and scissoring of the lower extremities, trunk arching. Poor suck-swallow, excessive drooling.

Diagnostic Studies: Karyotype for fragile X syndrome, fluorescent in situ hybridization (FISH), DNA probes. Magnetic resonance imaging (MRI) or CT scan.

Metabolic Studies: Ammonia level, liver function tests, electrolytes, total CO_2, venous blood gas level. Screen for amino acid and organic acid disorders. Organic acid assay, amino acid assay, mucopolysaccharides assay, enzyme deficiency assay.

Other Studies: Audiometry, free-thyroxine (T4), thyroid-stimulating hormone (TSH), blood lead levels, electrotromyography, nerve conduction velocities, muscle biopsy.

Differential Diagnosis of Developmental Delay

Static global delay/mental retardation
  Idiopathic mental retardation
  Chromosomal abnormalities or genetic syndromes
  Hypoxic-ischemic encephalopathy
  Structural brain malformation
  Prenatal exposure to toxins or teratogens
  Congenital infection
Progressive global delay
  Inborn errors of metabolism
  Neurodegenerative disorders
  Rett syndrome
  AIDS encephalopathy
  Congenital hypothyroidism
Language disorders
  Hearing impairment
  Language processing, expressive language disorders
  Pervasive developmental disorder or autistic disorder
Gross motor delay
  Cerebral palsy
  Peripheral neuromuscular disorders

Syndromes Associated With Development Delay
  Down Syndrome
  Fragile X Syndrome
  Prader-Willi Syndrome
  Turner Syndrome
  Williams Syndrome
  Noonan syndrome
  Sotos Syndrome
  Klinefelter Syndrome
  Angelman Syndrome
  Cornelia de Lange Syndrome
  Beckwith-Wiedemann Syndrome

Psychiatric History

I. **Identifying Information:** Age, gender.
II. **Chief Complaint:** Reason for the referral.
   A. **History of the Present Illness (HPI)**
      (1) **Developmental Level:** Cognitive, affective, interpersonal development.
      (2) **Neurodevelopmental Delay:** Cerebral palsy, mental retardation, congenital neurologic disorders.
      (3) **Organic Dysfunction:** Problems with perception, coordination, attention, learning, emotions, impulse control.
      (4) **Thought Disorders:** Delusions, hallucinations, disorganized speech, grossly disorganized or catatonic behavior, negative symptoms (eg, affective flattening, paucity of thought or speech).
      (5) **Anxiety and Behavioral Symptoms:** Phobias, obsessive-compulsive behaviors, depression.
      (6) **Temperamental Difficulty:** Adaptability, acceptability, demandingness.
      (7) **Psychophysiological Disorders:** Psychosomatic illnesses, conversion disorder.
      (8) **Unfavorable Environment:** Family or school problems.
      (9) **Causative Factors**
         a. **Genetic Disorders:** Dyslexia, attention-deficit hyperactivity disorder, mental retardation, autism.
         b. **Organic Disorders:** Malnutrition, intrauterine drug exposure, prematurity, head injury, central nervous system infections/tumors, metabolic conditions, toxins.
         c. **Developmental Delay:** Immaturity and attachment problems. Relationships with parents and siblings; developmental milestones, peer relationships, school performance
         d. **Inadequate Parenting:** Deprivation, separation, abuse, psychiatric disorders.
         e. **Stress Factors:** Illness, injury, surgery, hospitalizations, school failure, poverty.
         f. **Biological Function:** Appetite, sleep, bladder and bowel control, growth delay.
         g. **Relationships:** Family and peer problems.
         h. **Significant Life Events:** Separation and losses.
         i. **Previous Evaluations:** Previous psychiatric and neurological problems and assessments.
         j. **Parental Psychiatric State:** Status of each parent and their marriage. Relatives with psychiatric disorders, suicide, alcohol or substance abuse.
III. **Mental Status Examination**
   A. **Physical Appearance**
      (1) **Stature:** Age-appropriate appearance, precocity, head circumference.
      (2) **Dysmorphic Features:** Down syndrome, fragile X, fetal alcohol syndrome.
      (3) **Neurological Signs:** Weakness, cranial nerve palsies.
      (4) **Bruising:** Child abuse.
      (5) **Nutritional State:** Obesity, malnutrition, eating disorder.

- **(6) Movements:** Tics, biting of lips, hair pulling (ie, Tourette's disorder, anxiety).
- **(7) Spells:** Momentary lapses of attention, staring, head nodding, eye blinking (ie, epilepsy, hallucinations).
- **(8) Dress, Cleanliness, Hygiene:** Level of care and grooming.
- **(9) Mannerisms:** Thumb sucking, nail biting
- B. **Separation:** Excessive difficulty in separation.
- C. **Orientation**
    - **(1) To person:** Verbal children should know their names.
    - **(2) To place:** Young children should know whether they are away or at home.
    - **(3) To time:** A sense of time is formed by age 8 or 9. Young children can tell whether it is day or night.
- D. **Central Nervous System Function:** Soft signs (persistent neurodevelopmental immaturities):
    - **(1) Gross Motor Coordination Deficiency:** Impaired gait.
    - **(2) Fine Motor Coordination:** Copies a circle at age 2 to 3, cross at age 3 to 4, square at age 5, rhomboid at age 7.
        - **a. Laterality:** Right and left discrimination by age 5.
        - **b. Rapid Alternating Movements:** Hopping on one foot by age 7.
        - **c. Attention Span:** Distractibility, hyperactivity.
- E. **Reading or Writing Difficulties:** Dyslexia, dysgraphia.
- F. **Speech and Language Difficulties:** Autism, mental retardation, deprivation, regression.
- G. **Intelligence:** Vocabulary, level of comprehension, ability to identify body parts by age 5, drawing ability, mathematical ability.
- H. **Memory:** Children can count five digits forward and two backwards.
- I. **Thinking Process:** Logical and coherent thoughts, hallucinations, suicidal ideation, homicidal ideation, phobias, obsessions, delusions.
- J. **Fantasies and Inferred Conflicts:** Dreams, naming three wishes, drawing, spontaneous play.
- K. **Affect:** Anxiety, anger, depression, apathy.
- L. **Defense Organization:** Denial, projection, introversion, extroversion.
- M. **Judgment and Insight:** The child's opinion of the cause of the problem. How upset is the child about the problem?
- N. **Adaptive Capacities:** Problem-solving ability, resiliency.

Attempted Suicide and Drug Overdose

History of Present Illness: Time suicide was attempted and method. Quantity of pills; motive for attempt. Alcohol intake; where was substance obtained. Precipitating factor for suicide attempt (death, divorce, humiliating event); further desire to commit suicide. Is there a definite plan? Was the action impulsive or planned?

Feelings of sadness, guilt, hopelessness, helplessness. Reasons that the patient has to wish to go on living. Did the patient believe that he would succeed in suicide? Is the patient upset that he is still alive?

Past Psychiatric History: Previous suicide attempts or threats.

Medications: Antidepressants.

Family History: Depression, suicide, psychiatric disease, marital conflict, family support.

Social History: Personal or family history of emotional, physical, or sexual abuse; alcohol or drug abuse, sources of emotional stress. Availability of other dangerous medications or weapons.

Physical Examination

General Appearance: Level of consciousness, delirium; presence of potentially dangerous objects (belts, shoe laces).

Vital Signs: BP (hypotension), pulse (bradycardia), temperature, respiratory rate.

HEENT: Signs of trauma, ecchymoses; pupil size and reactivity, mydriasis, nystagmus.

Chest: Abnormal respiratory patterns, rhonchi (aspiration).

Heart: Arrhythmias, murmurs.

Abdomen: Decreased bowel sounds, tenderness.

Extremities: Wounds, ecchymoses, fractures.

Neurologic: Mental status exam; tremor, clonus, hyperactive reflexes.

Laboratory Evaluation: Electrolytes, BUN, creatinine, glucose. Alcohol, acetaminophen levels; chest X-ray, urine toxicology screen.

Toxicological Emergencies

History of Present Illness: Substance ingested, time of ingestion, quantity ingested (number of pills/volume of liquid). Was this a suicide attempt or gesture? Vomiting, lethargy, seizures, altered consciousness.

Past Medical History: Previous poisonings; heart, lung, kidney, gastrointestinal, or central nervous system disease.

Physical Examination

Vital Signs: Tachycardia (stimulants, anticholinergics), hypoventilation (narcotics, depressants), fever (anticholinergics, aspirin, stimulants).

Skin: Dry mucosa (anticholinergic); very moist skin (cholinergic or sympathomimetic).

Mouth:

Breath: Alcohol, hydrocarbon, cyanide odor.

Eyes: Meiosis, mydriasis, nystagmus (phenytoin or phencyclidine).

Chest: Breath sounds.

Cardiac: Bradycardia (beta-blocker, cholinergic, calcium channel blocker).

Abdomen: Decreased bowel sounds (anticholinergic or narcotic).

Neurological: Gait, reflexes, mental status, stimulation, sedation.

Laboratory Evaluation: Glucose (low in alcohols, oral hypoglycemics, aspirin, beta-blockers, insulin; high in iron, late aspirin), hypokalemia (lithium). Arterial blood gases. Liver function tests, WBC, toxicology screen of urine and serum. Methemoglobin test of blood. Ferric chloride urine test for aspirin.

Kidney, Ureter and Bladder (KUB) X-ray: Radiopaque pill fragments are seen with calcium, chloral hydrate, heavy metals (lead), iron, Pepto Bismol, phenothiazines, enteric-coated pills.

ECG: Prolonged QTc or widened QRS (tricyclic antidepressants).

Toxicologic Syndromes	
Toxin	**Clinical Findings**
Iron	Diarrhea, bloody stools, metabolic acidosis, hematemesis, coma, abdominal pain, leuko-cytosis, hyperglycemia
Opioids	Coma, respiratory depression, miosis, track marks, bradycardia, decreased bowel sounds
Organophosphates	Miosis, cramps, salivation, urination, broncho-rrhea, lacrimation, defecation, bradycardia
Salicylates	Hyperventilation, fever, diaphoresis, tinnitus, hypo- or hyperglycemia, hematemesis, altered mental status, metabolic acidosis, respiratory alkalosis
Phencyclidine (PCP)	Muscle twitching, rigidity, agitation, nystagmus, hypertension, tachycardia, psychosis, blank stare, myoglobinuria, increased creatinine phosphokinase
Tricyclic anti-depressants	Dry mucosa, vasodilation, hypotension, seizures, ileus, altered mental status, pupillary dilation, arrhythmias, widened QRS
Theophylline	Nausea, vomiting, tachycardia, tremor, convul-sions, metabolic acidosis, hypokalemia, ECG abnormalities
Adrenergic storm (cocaine, am-phetamines, phenylpropan-olamine)	Pupillary dilation, hyperthermia, agitation, diaphor-esis, seizures, tremor, anxiety, tactile hallucina-tions, dysrhythmias, active bowel sounds, track marks, hypertension
Sedative/hypnotics	Respiratory depression, coma, hypothermia, disconjugate eye movements
Anticholinergics	Dry mucous membranes and skin, tachycardia, fever, arrhythmias, urinary and fecal retention, mental status change, pupillary dilation, flushing

Trauma

History: Allergies, Medications, Past medical history, Last meal, and Events leading up to the injury (AMPLE). Determine the mechanism of injury and details of the trauma.

I. **Primary Survey: ABCDEs**
   A. **Airway:** Check for signs of obstruction (noisy breathing, inadequate air exchange). Normal speech indicates a patent airway.
   B. **Breathing:** Observe chest excursion. Auscultate chest.
   C. **Circulation:** Heart rate, blood pressure, pulse pressure, level of consciousness, capillary refill.
   D. **Disability**
      (1) **Level of Consciousness:** Alert, response to verbal stimuli, response to painful stimuli, unresponsive.
      (2) **Neurological Deficit:** Four extremity gross motor function, sensory deficits.
   E. **Exposure:** Completely undress the patient.

II. **Secondary Survey**
   A. **Head:** Raccoon eyes, Battle's sign, laceration, hematoma, deformity, skull fracture.
   B. **Face:** Laceration, deformity/asymmetry, bony tenderness.
   C. **Eyes:** Visual acuity, pupil reactivity, exothalmos, enophthalmos, hyphema, globe laceration, extraocular movements, lens dislocation.
   D. **Ears:** Laceration, hemotympanum, cerebrospinal fluid otorrhea.
   E. **Nose:** Laceration, nosebleed, septal hematoma, CSF rhinorrhea.
   F. **Mouth:** Lip laceration, tongue laceration, gum laceration, loose or missing teeth, foreign body, jaw tenderness/deformity.
   G. **Neck:** Laceration, hematoma, tracheal deviation, venous distention, carotid pulsation, cervical spine tenderness/deformity, tracheal deviation, subcutaneous emphysema, bruit, stridor.
   H. **Chest:** Symmetry, flail segments, laceration, rib and clavicle tenderness or deformity, subcutaneous emphysema, bilateral breath sounds, heart sounds.
   I. **Abdomen:** Laceration, ecchymosis, scars, tenderness, distention, bowel sounds, pelvis symmetry, deformity, tenderness, femoral pulse.
   J. **Rectal:** Sphincter tone, prostate position, occult blood.
   K. **Genitourinary:** Meatal blood, hematoma, laceration, tenderness, hematuria.
   L. **Extremities:** Color, deformity, laceration, hematoma, temperature, pulses, bony tenderness, capillary refill.
   M. **Back:** Ecchymosis, laceration, spine or rib tenderness, range of motion.
   N. **Neurological Examination:** Level of consciousness, pupil reactivity, sensation, reflexes, Babinski sign.

III. **Radiographic Evaluation of the Blunt Trauma Patient**
   A. **Standard trauma series**
      (1) Cervical spine
      (2) Chest X ray
      (3) Pelvic radiograph
      (4) Computed Tomography (CT)

Commonly Used Abbreviations

½ NS	0.45% saline solution	CO_2	carbon dioxide
ac	ante cibum (before meals)	COPD	chronic obstructive pulmonary disease
ABG	arterial blood gas	CPK-MB	myocardial-specific CPK isoenzyme
ac	before meals		
ACTH	adrenocorticotropic hormone	CPR	cardiopulmonary resuscitation
ad lib	ad libitum (desired)	CSF	cerebrospinal fluid
ADH	antidiuretic hormone	CT	computerized tomography
AFB	acid-fast bacillus	CVP	central venous pressure
alk phos	alkaline phosphatase	CXR	Chest X-ray
ALT	alanine amino-transferase	d/c	discharge; discontinue
		D5W	5% dextrose water solution; also D10W, D50W
am	morning		
AMA	against medical advice	DIC	disseminated intravascular coagulation
amp	ampule		
AMV	assisted mandatory ventilation; assist mode ventilation	diff	differential count
		DKA	diabetic ketoacidosis
		dL	deciliter
ANA	antinuclear antibody	DOSS	docusate sodium sulfosuccinate
ante	before		
AP	anteroposterior	DTs	delirium tremens
ARDS	adult respiratory distress syndrome	ECG	electrocardiogram
		ER	emergency room
ASA	acetylsalicylic acid	ERCP	endoscopic retrograde cholangiopancreatography
AST	aspartate amino-transferase		
		ESR	erythrocyte sedimentation rate
bid	bis in die (twice a day)		
B-12	vitamin B-12 (cyanocobalamin)	ET	endotracheal tube
		ETOH	alcohol
BM	bowel movement	FEV_1	forced expiratory volume (in one second)
BP	blood pressure		
BUN	blood urea nitrogen	FiO2	fractional inspired oxygen
c/o	complaint of	g	gram(s)
c̄	cum (with)	GC	gonococcal; gonococcus
C and S	culture and sensitivity	GFR	glomerular filtration rate
C	centigrade	GI	gastrointestinal
Ca	calcium	gm	gram
cap	capsule	gt	drop
CBC	complete blood count; includes hemoglobin, hematocrit, red blood cell indices, white blood cell count, and platelets	gtt	drops
		h	hour
		H_2O	water
		HBsAG	hepatitis B surface antigen
		HCO_3	bicarbonate
cc	cubic centimeter	Hct	hematocrit
CCU	coronary care unit	HDL	high-density lipoprotein
cm	centimeter	Hg	mercury
CMF	cyclophosphamide, methotrexate, fluorouracil	Hgb	hemoglobin concentration
		HIV	human immunodeficiency virus
CNS	central nervous system	hr	hour

hs	hora somni (bedtime, hour of sleep)	NKA	no known allergies
IM	intramuscular	NPH	neutral protamine Hagedorn (insulin)
I and O	intake and output--measurement of the patient's intake and output	NPO	nulla per os (nothing by mouth)
IU	international units	NS	normal saline solution (0.9%)
ICU	intensive care unit	NSAID	nonsteroidal anti-inflammatory drug
IgM	immunoglobulin M		
IMV	intermittent mandatory ventilation	O_2	oxygen
		OD	right eye
INH	isoniazid	oint	ointment
INR	International normalized ratio	OS	left eye
		Osm	osmolality
IPPB	intermittent positive-pressure breathing	OT	occupational therapy
		OTC	over the counter
IV	intravenous or intravenously	OU	each eye
		oz	ounce
IVP	intravenous pyelogram; intravenous piggyback	p, post	after
		pc	post cibum (after meals)
K^+	potassium	PA	posteroanterior; pulmonary artery
kcal	kilocalorie		
KCL	potassium chloride	PaO_2	arterial oxygen pressure
KPO_4	potassium phosphate	pAO_2	partial pressure of oxygen in alveolar gas
KUB	x-ray of abdomen (kidneys, ureters, bowels)		
		PB	phenobarbital
L	liter	pc	after meals
LDH	lactate dehydrogenase	$pCO2$	partial pressure of carbon dioxide
LDL	low-density lipoprotein		
liq	liquid	PEEP	positive end-expiratory pressure
LLQ	left lower quadrant		
LP	lumbar puncture, low potency	per	by
		pH	hydrogen ion concentration (H+)
LR	lactated Ringer's (solution)		
		PID	pelvic inflammatory disease
MB	myocardial band	pm	afternoon
MBC	minimal bacterial concentration	PO	orally, per os
		pO_2	partial pressure of oxygen
mcg	microgram	polys	polymorphonuclear leukocytes
mEq	milliequivalent		
mg	milligram	PPD	purified protein derivative
Mg	magnesium	PR	per rectum
$MgSO_4$	Magnesium Sulfate	prn	pro re nata (as needed)
MI	myocardial infarction	PT	physical therapy; prothrombin time
MIC	minimum inhibitory concentration		
		PTCA	percutaneous transluminal coronary angioplasty
mL	milliliter		
mm	millimeter	PTT	partial thromboplastin time
MOM	Milk of Magnesia	PVC	premature ventricular contraction
MRI	magnetic resonance imaging		
		q	quaque (every) q6h, q2h every 6 hours; every 2 hours
Na	sodium		
$NaHCO_3$	sodium bicarbonate	qid	quarter in die (four times a day)
Neuro	neurologic		
NG	nasogastric	qAM	every morning

qd	quaque die (every day)	TPA	tissue plasminogen activator
qh	every hour	TSH	thyroid-stimulating hormone
qhs	every night before bedtime	tsp	teaspoon
		U	units
qid	4 times a day	UA	urinalysis
qOD	every other day	URI	upper respiratory infection
qs	quantity sufficient	Ut Dict	as directed
R/O	rule out	UTI	urinary tract infection
RA	rheumatoid arthritis; room air; right atrial	VAC	vincristine, adriamycin, and cyclophosphamide
Resp	respiratory rate	vag	vaginal
RL	Ringer's lactated solution (also LR)	VC	vital capacity
		VDRL	Venereal Disease Research Laboratory
ROM	range of motion	VF	ventricular function
rt	right	V fib	ventricular fibrillation
s	sine (without)	VLDL	very low-density lipoprotein
s/p	status post	Vol	volume
sat	saturated	VS	vital signs
SBP	systolic blood pressure	VT	ventricular tachycardia
SC	subcutaneously	W	water
SIADH	syndrome of inappropriate antidiuretic hormone	WBC	white blood count
		x	times
SL	sublingually under tongue		
SLE	systemic lupus erythematosus		
SMA-12	sequential multiple analysis; a panel of 12 chemistry tests. Tests include Na$^+$, K$^+$, HCO3 , chloride, BUN, glucose, creatinine, bilirubin, calcium, total protein, albumin, alkaline phosphatase.		
SMX	sulfamethoxazole		
sob	shortness of breath		
sol	solution		
SQ	under the skin		
ss	one-half		
STAT	statim (immediately)		
susp	suspension		
tid	ter in die (three times a day)		
T4	Thyroxine level (T4)		
tab	tablet		
TB	tuberculosis		
Tbsp	tablespoon		
Temp	temperature		
TIA	transient ischemic attack		
tid	three times a day		
TKO	to keep open, an infusion rate (500 mL/24h)		
TMP-SMX	trimethoprim-sulfamethoxazole combination		

Index

Titles from Current Clinical Strategies Publishing

In All Medical Bookstores Worldwide

Family Medicine, 2000 Edition
Outpatient Medicine, 2001 Edition
History and Physical Examination, 2001-2002 Edition
Medicine, 2001Edition
Pediatrics 5 Minute Review, 1998-99 Edition
Anesthesiology, 1999-2000 Edition
Handbook of Psychiatric Drugs, 2002 Edition
Gynecology and Obstetrics, 1999-2000 Edition
Manual of HIV/AIDS Therapy, 2001 Edition
Practice Parameters in Medicine and Primary Care, 1999-2000
  Edition
Surgery, 1999-2000 Edition
Pediatric Drug Reference, 2000 Edition
Critical Care Medicine, 2000 Edition
Psychiatry, 1999-2000 Edition
Pediatrics, 2000 Edition
Physicians' Drug Resource, 1999 Edition
Pediatric History and Physical Examination, Fourth Edition

CD-ROM and Softcover Book